The Solution
Focused
Brief Therapy
Diamond

◆

Praise for
THE SOLUTION FOCUSED BRIEF THERAPY DIAMOND

This is a love story, a book about love. Love for clients, love for each other and love for solution focused brief therapy.

Elliott and Adam pour out their hearts to each other and to us in this story of a relationship that might change the world.

If anyone has said the solution focused approach is lacking in emotion, they should read this book for within it they will find the heart and soul of the kindest therapeutic model ever created.

Elliott and Adam teach us more how-to-be than how-to-do. The how-to-do solution focused brief therapy is there, but it lies within a more important context of how-to-be.

Chapter by chapter, Elliott 'dives deep' looking for the emotional glue that holds the model together, while Adam 'takes a closer look' at the language of solution focused brief therapy and how this, too, holds the model together. Through this process they chart new territory and very new ways of thinking about and doing therapy. It is one of the triumphs of this book that when it comes to the doing or practice of solution focused brief therapy, Elliott and Adam have kept it simple, perhaps the simplest version so far. The 'Diamond' is an easy-to-follow guideline for conducting a solution focused therapy session. Though much of what the originators of the approach, Steve de Shazer and Insoo Kim Berg, advocated has been uncompromisingly stripped out, Adam and Elliott have stayed absolutely true to its central tenets: that the client is the expert, description is the driver of change and everything therapists do should be tested for its validity.

Elliott and Adam have created a 'bible' for the next decade of solution focused brief therapy. They have gone far beyond yet stayed totally true to technique. It will be a primary text for beginners and a creative challenge to even the most experienced solution focused practitioners. This book represents a new coming-of-age for the entire solution focused field and like solution focused brief therapy itself it is both a labour of great love and a work of art.

— **Chris Iveson**, SFBT practitioner and trainer and co-founder of BRIEF

◆

The Solution
Focused
Brief Therapy
Diamond

A New Approach to SFBT That Will
Empower Both Practitioner and Client
to Achieve the Best Outcomes

ELLIOTT E. CONNIE AND ADAM S. FROERER

HAY HOUSE

Carlsbad, California • New York City
London • Sydney • New Delhi

Published in the United Kingdom by:

Hay House UK Ltd, The Sixth Floor, Watson House,

54 Baker Street, London W1U 7BU

Tel: +44 (0)20 3927 7290; Fax: +44 (0)20 3927 7291; www.hayhouse.co.uk

Published in the United States of America by:

Hay House Inc., PO Box 5100, Carlsbad, CA 92018-5100

Tel: (1) 760 431 7695 or (800) 654 5126

Fax: (1) 760 431 6948 or (800) 650 5115; www.hayhouse.com

Published in Australia by:

Hay House Australia Ltd, 18/36 Ralph St, Alexandria NSW 2015

Tel: (61) 2 9669 4299; Fax: (61) 2 9669 4144; www.hayhouse.com.au

Published in India by:

Hay House Publishers India, Muskaan Complex, Plot No.3, B-2,

Vasant Kunj, New Delhi 110 070

Tel: (91) 11 4176 1620; Fax: (91) 11 4176 1630; www.hayhouse.co.in

Project editor: Melody Guy • *Indexer:* Jay Kreider • *Cover design:* Jason Gabbert
Interior design: Bryn Starr Best • *Illustration:* ©2021 Elliott Connie & Adam Froerer

A catalogue record for this book is available from the British Library.

Tradepaper ISBN: 978-1-78817-849-5
E-book ISBN: 978-1-4019-7050-5
Audiobook ISBN: 978-1-4019-7051-2

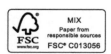

We dedicate this book to all the people
who have inspired us to inspire others.

This book is for each of the clients who
helped us understand the power of this approach.
Thank you for helping us perceive the details and for
helping us be in awe of the transformation we
are each capable of achieving!

◇◇

What outcome do you want from reading this book?

_____

_____

_____

_____

What difference would it make if you could attain it?

_____

_____

_____

_____

How would you notice the change it made in your life?

_____

_____

_____

_____

◇◇

Contents

PART IV: BEYOND THE BASICS

Introduction

Love! This book is a labor of love. This is a book about our love for solution focused brief therapy (SFBT), even to the smallest detail. But more importantly, this book is a book about how doing SFBT must happen from a place of love. We would go so far as to say that we need to love our clients. We know this isn't a typical way to start a book, nor is this a typical way to frame an entire book. We know we are bucking all the formal teaching about psychotherapy that encourages clinicians to keep a healthy distance between clients and themselves.

Now, we aren't encouraging clinicians to be unethical or to act inappropriately, but we are encouraging mental health professionals to rethink the way they approach their work. We are asking professionals to reevaluate the stance they take when encountering individuals, couples, and families who are experiencing hardship. We are promising that this book can change your professional life (and potentially your personal life) if you work from the innovative place of love!

This book is divided into four sections. Part I begins by looking at the evolution of SFBT and how we developed the diamond model. This evolution begins with the love story between Steve and Insoo (shared with us by Insoo's daughter, Sarah). The book then progresses with an ongoing emphasis on overcoming differences to find strength and innovation.

Part I concludes with our own stories and how we came to be leaders within the solution focused field. These stories highlight experiences we've had that have taught us the importance of working from a place of love and respect. We highlight how overcoming discrimination and other challenges have paved the way for conceptualizing the solution focused approach in this unique, evolved way.

Part II outlines the stance of effective solution focused clinicians. We cover how SFBT clinicians can ADOPT (stay tuned for more explanation about this) a loving stance of viewing and appreciating others that will change the course of their clinical work. This stance-description is followed in Part III by a detailed description of the SFBT diamond model. The diamond model is outlined in precise detail and is supplemented with actual case examples to bring the nuts and bolts to life. This is the most comprehensive overview of the evolved SFBT approach to date.

Finally, Part IV provides additional tools to help you find success in implementing this approach. There are three appendices as well: The first is a document with 101 SFBT questions, categorized to reflect the diamond model, which serves as a reference guide for all clinicians. The second is a complete session with editorial comments that illustrate the thinking that goes into constructing SFBT sessions. Rarely can you find a session with such detailed analysis in all SFBT literature. The third is a glossary that defines key SFBT terms. We hope these tools provide practical help for all clinicians working within the diamond framework.

Each chapter is structured in an atypical manner. We (Elliott and Adam) are quite different from one another and often have very different perspectives and styles when it comes to the explanation of what we are seeing in solution focused work. To capture our individual styles and voices, we have included smaller sections within each chapter that are entitled "Diving Deep with Elliott" and "A Closer Look with Adam." These sections aren't meant to be contradictory or confusing, but rather they are meant to show that we can have different but complementary perspectives that when woven together make our appreciation for the approach even richer. We hope that you will consider both perspectives equally and that you will feel free to add your own perspective. As we mention in the book, it is because of our differences that the SFBT diamond model works so well. We hope your own understanding of the solution focused approach is enhanced because of our unique perspectives.

We encourage you to use this book in any way that is useful to you. You may find that reading the book straight through makes the most sense. We have written the book in a way that builds, chapter by chapter, to create a clear understanding of how we approach our work. However, you will likely find that referencing a specific chapter to gain more clarity and understanding will be useful, as each part and chapter can stand alone. We imagine that some clinicians will want to mark certain things and come back to those over and over. We know in our own work that re-referencing important components or thoughts has been really helpful. We hope this book will be that reference point for you. Finally, it is possible that some people will combine these two approaches, sometimes focusing on the technical components and sometimes looking for encouragement through the personal stories. However you decide to use the book, we hope it will meet your needs, which will likely change over time. Use the book in the way that makes the most sense to you.

In whatever way you choose to use the book, we hope that you walk away feeling inspired. We hope this book increases your ability to view people as strong, capable, and resilient. We hope this book enhances your ability to co-construct solution focused conversations with your clients and with other people in your life. We hope you walk away feeling an increased sense of love for your work, for the solution focused diamond model, and for the people you work with. Of course we hope you feel more competent and capable of having solution focused conversations, but most importantly, we hope you feel the love that we intended to pass to you through these pages. Thank you for allowing us to be a small part of your journey to excellence!

PART I

An Introduction to Solution Focused Brief Therapy

Chapter 1

Solution Focused Brief Therapy

An Evolutionary Approach

Stop the Old Way of Thinking

Clear your mind before you read this book. Within its pages, you'll learn our unique approach to solution focused brief therapy (SFBT), an evidence-based form of psychotherapy that helps people create change in their lives. But before you do that, we need you to stop thinking like a therapist. We need to engage with you, the individual, not the psychotherapy version of you. The truth is you already know how to practice SFBT. It's inherent. It's about agency, something you're already well versed in.

Think about the parents of young children—parents who are perfectly capable of tying their children's shoes. The task isn't difficult. It's also a more efficient way to get the family out the door on time. But as children get older, parents choose to let them tie their own shoes. They understand that agency is important in terms of skill acquisition. In order to raise children who can accomplish tasks on their own, parents have to refrain from doing tasks for them, even though helping them is the quickest solution in the moment.

That's solution focused brief therapy in a nutshell. It is connecting with the version of your client (or anyone in your life) that you want to talk to, the version that fundamentally understands the importance of autonomy.

As a therapist, you went to school and learned a collection of techniques that were supposed to assist you in helping a client. But SFBT techniques are completely different. They involve facilitating a conversation that will honor client agency and lead toward change in a different manner.

You can't learn this approach by thinking in the old way. It's too different from other methods that define therapists as people whose job it is to change their clients.

Again, clear your mind—even when it comes to preconceptions you may have about solution focused brief therapy. To begin with, it's not a name that we would have chosen, but it's the name our field has adopted. Consequently, although misleading, it's the name we're stuck with.

Solution focused brief therapy implies we're meant to solve something and find solutions for our clients. Instead we're meant to build something and construct change with them.

It's not our job to fix them. It's our job to inspire, to connect, and to help them describe the outcomes they desire, then watch what happens in the process.

In this book, we'll share exactly how to do that.

A Brief History of SFBT

Solution focused brief therapy (SFBT) is a therapeutic approach that is focused on where the client would like to end up, rather than focusing on problem(s) and problem development, as many other therapeutic approaches do. This outcome-focused approach was a paradigm shift at its founding and still challenges the status quo of psychotherapy today. The seeds of solution focused brief therapy started at the Mental Research Institute (MRI) in Palo Alto, California, where psychotherapists Steve de Shazer and Insoo Kim Berg met. They dated, subsequently married, and moved to

Wisconsin, where they created the Brief Family Therapy Center in Milwaukee in 1978.

Steve and Insoo's focus was on making therapy briefer. At the time, psychotherapy was synonymous with psychoanalysis, which involved a client coming to therapy two to three times a week for three to five years. Steve and Insoo, along with the MRI team, asked themselves one basic question: Can we make therapy briefer without sacrificing outcomes? The MRI team was able to reduce the average number of sessions down to about 10, a significant decrease from the traditional psychodynamic approach.

Later, from the research conducted at the Brief Family Therapy Center in Milwaukee, Steve and Insoo developed solution focused brief therapy. Using this approach, they were able to reduce the number of times a client came to therapy from even MRI's standard of 10 sessions, while still being just as effective at impacting a client's problem.

That's where the solution focused approach sprouted, and from there it branched out. One large branch developed in London in the 1990s and early 2000s at BRIEF, an independent training, therapy, and consultation agency for SFBT. The BRIEF team in London—Chris Iveson, Harvey Ratner, and Evan George—took the Milwaukee approach, but they wanted to see if they could make it even briefer.

In the same vein, we have taken the BRIEF approach and aimed to make it even briefer, something we refer to as "straightening the line," or in other words making therapy as efficient as possible. We created The Solution Focused Universe, a worldwide training institute, and developed one of the largest current contributions in our field, the diamond model to SFBT. We believe our diamond model is the straightest line possible with SFBT. So in an evolutionary manner, there's a connection from MRI to Steve and Insoo to BRIEF to us.

A Perpetually Evolutionary Approach

A Closer Look with Adam

One of the major premises of solution focused brief therapy, which Steve and Insoo established early on, is the concept that, if what you're doing as a therapist is working, do more of it, and if it isn't, do something different.

Following that line of thinking, Elliott and I also view our work as open to evolution. Our approach is built on Steve and Insoo's foundation, but it's also inherently different, which is the rationale for the diamond model.

In our field, there's a debate between purists and evolutionists. Should therapists practice SFBT exactly as Steve and Insoo first laid it out 40 years ago, or can we appreciate that they themselves were proponents of change?

They took psychotherapy and flipped it upside down and said that, instead of focusing on the problem or diagnosis or being reductionistic in how to view people, they were going to go about their work in a different way. The fact that they were evolutionary is an argument that we should continue to be evolutionary. Our diamond model is a result of that evolution.

Along with the mechanics of the diamond, what really sets our approach apart is its stance—the position we take about viewing our clients as capable and strong and worthy collaborators in co-constructing effective therapy.

I believe Steve and Insoo would have bought into that stance, though they didn't talk about it overtly. They took for granted that therapists should feel that way about people. And because they didn't talk about it, falsehoods have been perpetuated.

People mischaracterize Steve's words when they say, "We don't need to worry about the therapeutic alliance," meaning clinicians don't need to pay special consideration to the relationship between the client and the therapist.

I doubt he meant we don't need to attend to it; I just think he assumed that we already did, or that doing so would involve new mindsets beyond those that therapists typically have for their clients—mindsets that came naturally to Steve and Insoo.

Adopting that mindset (the stance) of seeing a client as a strong and capable person, and as a worthwhile contributor, is something Elliott and I go out of our way to advocate. Therapists must take that stance toward their clients because it impacts the way they work together. If that stance is neglected, a therapist's work isn't going to be sufficient.

While the stance isn't necessarily evolutionary, it's something that hasn't been emphasized in the past. Elliott has many stories about how he has been mistreated in this field, and he and I have come to emphasize what we emphasize because of his experience as a person of color.

As an Asian woman, Insoo was also a person of color, but she was working in this field 40 years ago. Whereas in this moment in time—a post–George Floyd era—we have to be overt about the stance, which is that we see each client as unique and specifically valuable. I'm confident Steve or Insoo would agree, but they weren't having that conversation in the late '70s and early '80s. Today that conversation is essential.

There's a political intersection, a time-period intersection, and a racial intersection that we have to consider as we practice psychotherapy now, as well as how each of those have evolved over the past few decades. We also need to take into account how worldviews and globalization play a role. As therapists, our methods and mindsets must evolve and become relevant to this day and age.

That perspective falls right in line with another major premise of SFBT, also outlined by Steve and Insoo, which is the importance of being thoughtful and consistent about language.

All in all, SFBT hasn't really changed over the years as much as the language we need to use about it has—language that first and foremost pays respect to our clients by maximizing their agency as we co-construct a meaningful therapy session with them. In this book, we'll teach you exactly how to do that.

An Approach Based on Love, Connection, and Acceptance

Diving Deep with Elliott

In many respects, solution focused brief therapy is counterintuitive, whereas the much more common approach of cognitive behavioral therapy is linear and logical.

Let's say a client comes to you with a problem like heroin addiction. Overcoming that addiction in a rapid manner doesn't make logical sense, but I have videotaped sessions of heroin-addicted clients who transformed quickly during SFBT work with me.

When I started my teaching career, I didn't share any of those videos, and people didn't believe my claims about the effectiveness of SFBT. I was young at the time, and more experienced therapists rebuffed me, saying that in over 30 years of experience in their own respective practices, they never saw clients change as rapidly as I alleged that mine did.

When I began showing videos, they finally started believing my words. The evidence was right in front of them.

SFBT is a powerful approach that cuts right through to the heart of what people really need. When they feel loved, connected, and accepted, they're truly capable of anything.

Love. Connection. Acceptance. It's as simple as that.

Instead, therapists tend to complicate matters. They want to figure out what's wrong with their clients so they can fix it. What if they shifted their way of thinking? What if you did? What if instead of trying to figure out the root of your clients' problems, you learned to accept them, despite their issues? What if you learned how to love on them? Connect with them?

In my experience, that's how clients get better.

Taking that stance became my motivator, the thing that drove me.

Open your mind to it. Let it drive you too.

Chapter 2

Steve de Shazer and Insoo Kim Berg

A Love Story and Legacy

Believe in Miracles

The solution focused approach began in the most fitting way possible—with a love story. Its founders, Steve de Shazer and Insoo Kim Berg, came together as a couple 40 years ago, and 40 years later their relationship and legacy continue to inspire those in our field.

Both Steve and Insoo were psychotherapists. Steve was from Milwaukee, Wisconsin, and Insoo was from Korea but immigrated to Milwaukee. That's not where the two of them met, however.

Steve found his way to Palo Alto, California, and was training at the Mental Research Institute (MRI), where other therapists were doing pioneering work in systemic approaches to the helping professions, including working with families and focusing on communication.

The MRI became a remarkable place in our field. So many cutting-edge ideas were developed and experimented upon there, spearheaded by leading figures in psychotherapy such as Paul Watzlawick, John Weakland, Jay Haley, Don D. Jackson, and the list goes on.

Insoo also went to the MRI to receive training, and that's where she met Steve. On the surface, the two of them had nothing in common—nothing that would have initially attracted them as a couple other than their shared interest in effective modalities of therapy.

After Insoo completed her training and moved back to Milwaukee, she continued to travel back to the MRI every three to four months and stay for one or two days of additional training. Over time, the frequency with which she traveled to California started increasing. Why? She began pursuing Steve.

According to Sarah Kim Berg, Insoo's daughter from her first marriage, Insoo gravitated to Steve not because of an initial physical attraction but because she was deeply attracted to his mind.

Steve was very bright and a deep thinker, and as Insoo shared her thoughts with him, "talking in circles" at times, he would take it all in, listening intently, and then express what she'd said back to her in beautiful and succinct sentences.

He had a gift for understanding what she was saying and synthesizing it, which enamored her, and from that place of being captivated, a relationship grew—so much so that Insoo persuaded him to move back to Milwaukee.

There they married and decided to create the "MRI of the Midwest," trying to replicate what was being done in Palo Alto. But they made one change: they stopped telling their clients how many sessions they were going to have. This was a departure from the MRI's standard practice of giving each client 10 sessions.

Insoo noticed that when clients were told they had 10 sessions, they tended to use all of them. They didn't start working hard until the seventh or eighth session. But when they didn't know how many sessions they had to work with, clients began the change process much sooner.

This was the first modification that led to what we now know as solution focused brief therapy.

In 1978, Steve and Insoo co-founded the Brief Family Therapy Center (BFTC) in Milwaukee, where their group of therapists saw cases as a team. While one conducted a session with a client, the others watched behind a one-way mirror. The purpose was to identify and understand what was working in their approach so they could do more of it.

On top of that, Steve and Insoo often conducted therapy at their home and invited therapists to come and observe their sessions. Imagine how remarkable it would have been to sit on their staircase, with a view into their living room, and observe their work—the work of two world-renowned therapists—and afterward be able to give them feedback.

The beginning of solution focused brief therapy was beautifully simple and organic in that way. At its heart were just two people who had fallen in love and committed to working together and building a team that could continue to find out what was truly effective in psychotherapy.

SFBT started out as an experiment. Its aim was to figure out what makes change happen and how therapists can be more efficient with people's time, all while helping them create lasting change in the most simple and direct way possible.

Understanding the original ideas and the original foundation of the solution focused approach is important so therapists can always draw inspiration from those beginnings and never forget where they have come from as solution focused professionals.

We had the great pleasure of meeting Sarah Kim Berg in the spring of 2021. She was unbelievably giving with her time as she toured us around sites in Milwaukee, such as the first location of BFTC, Steve and Insoo's home, and even their final resting place, which couldn't have been easy for her.

When we asked Sarah what had prompted her to be so generous, she said, "My mother would have loved your work and the two of you working together."

That really touched us because, like Steve and Insoo, we are very different but work together magically, and to think that Insoo would have recognized that in us is very special.

Also like Steve and Insoo, we care deeply about people. We're trying to change the world by teaching therapists how to help one person at a time.

The stance that Steve and Insoo took about their relationship, their clients, and their life can be summed up best by the powerful yet simple mantra engraved on their shared headstone: Believe in miracles.

Insoo's Journey to Freedom

Insoo never talked about her childhood or how hard it was to be a teenager in Korea during the Korean War. Sarah learned what she relayed to us through her aunt, Insoo's sister.

Insoo's father worked for the Korean government and was wanted by the North Koreans as a political prisoner. He left home to hide from them, and the family didn't know where he was, if he was alive, or when he'd be able to return.

Insoo's mother was interrogated and threatened frequently by the North Koreans, who demanded to know the whereabouts of her husband. Worried about the safety of her children, she sent three of them away—Insoo, who was the oldest, and her two younger brothers. Her mother would remain home with her youngest child, Insoo's sister, who was too little to make the journey.

At about 16 years of age, Insoo was given the huge task of leaving Seoul and walking her younger brothers to the southern coast of South Korea, a journey of hundreds of miles, and taking them to safety.

She had no supplies, and her country was at war, but she managed to find food along the way and ultimately arrived at their destination. It wasn't until later in life that she would finally be reunited with her mom and younger sister.

When Sarah told us this story, it was like a lightbulb flashed on for us. Suddenly Insoo's tenacious nature in her career made perfect sense.

Of course she would go on to create an approach that was about an outcome, because as a 16-year-old she was focused on arriving at an outcome herself—freedom. It didn't matter how far she and her brothers had to walk or if it was cold or how old they were.

Of course she would develop an approach that doesn't attend to obstacles but instead focuses on destinations.

Of course she would advocate for therapy that aimed at taking one step at a time, because how else can you walk hundreds of miles to find safety from war?

When people claim that SFBT is about positivity, we argue, "No, it's about determination." You have to be very determined and focused to do what Insoo did at 16 years old.

Is it really surprising then that someone like her could live the rest of her life thinking, *People can do anything?*

Where did she find that determination and inspiration? Where can you? The answer lies in the past, in your own history of resilience and success. Each of us has made our own journeys. Each of us has crossed figurative borders. Harnessing those victories is the magic of this approach.

If you can remember the obstacles you've conquered, then when clients tell you about their own obstacles, it will be easy for you to be like Insoo and think, *You can get through this. You can achieve anything.*

Why I Chose to Practice Solution Focused Brief Therapy

Diving Deep with Elliott

When I went to graduate school, I thought psychotherapy was just a job. I didn't know different forms of psychotherapy were still being practiced, driven by various theories. I thought it evolved like technology, in the same way eight-track players phased out record players, which were then replaced by cassette players, CD players, MP3 players, and eventually streaming platforms.

Along those lines, I thought psychotherapy evolved from Sigmund Freud to Carl Jung to Alfred Adler and so on. Halfway through graduate school, I worked at a job where everyone practiced cognitive behavioral therapy, so I assumed it was the latest approach—what the whole field was practicing—as well as what I'd go on to learn about in school. I didn't realize there were other options.

In one of my courses, my class studied from a book in which every chapter highlighted a different theory of psychotherapy. A thrill of excitement ran through me as I opened to the first chapter. I was finally going to learn some practical application.

Chapter 1 discussed Sigmund Freud, including the Oedipus complex and his theories and methods of psychoanalysis. When I finished reading that chapter, I felt relieved and comforted. A really smart person had just explained to me how people change. Awesome.

The next week, I read Chapter 2, which was about Carl Jung, who essentially said, "I agree with Freud about these things, but I disagree about these other things. Consequently, I've created something called Jungian therapy, which is about the collective unconscious and analyzing the 'real' self."

Unease stirred within me. There were now two competing thoughts about how people change.

During the third week, I read Chapter 3, which was about Alfred Adler and his Adlerian therapy, focusing on the development of individual personality while also encouraging a sense of belonging.

Now there were three competing thoughts on how people change. I grew frustrated. I just wanted to be told how to practice psychotherapy in the best way.

I eventually completed the course and got an A in the class, but all the while I kept thinking, *How am I supposed to do my job?*

The next semester I took a class about family therapy approaches, which are different in nature and are referred to as systemic. *Okay*, I thought. *I'm going to learn how to work with families.* But I came up against the same roadblock: chapter after chapter of conflicting approaches.

My frustration rooted deeper. At that time of my life, the only skill I had a real talent for was playing baseball. Now let's say I had gone to college to learn how to hit a baseball, but what I was taught instead was who invented the game, who invented the baseball bat, and what different theories existed for baseball swings. Those wouldn't help me. What would help is being taught the mechanics of hitting a baseball. I wanted that same help with psychotherapy, but nothing in graduate school was fitting the bill.

I really can't overstate my frustration. I wasn't in graduate school for the same reasons as my peers. Most of them wanted to be psychotherapists or wanted a master's degree or to receive a Ph.D. because they realized medical school wasn't for them. Not me. I didn't give a damn about the degree on the wall. I didn't care what the job was called. I was in graduate school for one reason, and that was to help people. But I didn't feel like I was learning how to do that, even though I was paying a lot of money.

I had a professor by the name of Dr. Ronnie McManus, and if you look up "professor" in the dictionary, you'll see a picture of him. He was a tall guy with a long gray beard and eyes filled with gentleness. The quintessential professor. If I could cast a professor in a movie, I would cast Dr. Ronnie McManus circa 2005.

One day after class, I said to him, "You've got to help me. I'm thinking about quitting school because I'm not learning the mechanics of how to do this job. I'm just learning theory and history."

I'll never forget how he smiled, put his hand on my shoulder, and replied, "Elliott, you have to ask yourself, *How do you think people learn?*"

Although Dr. McManus had spoken as warmly and kindly as a person could, I viewed his answer as unsatisfactory.

As I drove home, white-knuckling the steering wheel in sheer aggravation, I finally took my professor's words to heart. *"Okay, Elliott,"* I asked myself, *"how do you learn?"*

I thought back on how I'd learned to hit a baseball, and I remembered my high school baseball coach, Peter Pasquarosa, whom my team and I called "Coach P."

Coach P did something in 1993–1994 that was groundbreaking, although I didn't realize it then. He would videotape our baseball team during batting practice. Each player would get about 15 swings, and the next day before practice we would go into a class-room together and Coach P would play the tape for us.

One day as we were watching the video, he only played 3 of my 15 swings. I asked why, and he answered, "I picked your three best swings because those are the ones I want you to repeat."

Now think about what he had to do every day to show us our best swings. Today, editing video isn't difficult, so it has become more common for coaches to do what Coach P did back then. But editing video almost 30 years ago was very laborious, and Coach P was doing it for his *entire* baseball team—editing his recordings to only show us our best swings.

Over my high school years, he helped me become a better baseball player, and he did it without ever highlighting my mistakes. He wasn't the type of guy who asked you to fix problems; he asked you to repeat brilliance.

As I reflected on this, I asked myself, *Is there an approach to psychotherapy that's in line with Coach P's method?*

I also thought about my own life story, much of which had been very painful. If I'd had to meet with a therapist, sit down with him, and tell him about my past, it would have caused me emotional injury.

I don't believe I'm rare in that sense. Recently, Adam and I went on a trip to the American South and interviewed people who were involved in the civil rights movement. We met a guy named Hezekiah Watkins, who had been the youngest Freedom Rider at 13 years old during the Freedom Rides, a series of political protests against racial segregation on buses in 1961.

When we interviewed Hezekiah, we said, "Can we ask you questions about what it was like to be a Freedom Rider?"

"Of course you can," he replied. "But please don't ask me what it was like to be on death row."

Most of the Freedom Riders spent the summer of 1961 in the Mississippi State Penitentiary, also known as Parchman prison, and Hezekiah was put on death row for five days until the governor of Mississippi ordered his release.

Sixty years later, Hezekiah told us, "I'm still not able to talk about death row without suffering."

He knew his boundaries, and as an almost 30-year-old graduate student, I knew mine. As I examined how I learned in the best way possible, at the urging of Dr. Ronnie McManus, I understood that learning by invoking suffering wasn't something I believed in. Instead, I believed that people learned by analyzing their brilliance.

Again, the only effective psychotherapy approach that fell in line for me was solution focused brief therapy—the only approach that didn't require the client to suffer. That's what hooked me.

SFBT isn't about minimizing problems. We know they're real and true and people have them. However, in spite of problems, people find remarkable ways to achieve brilliance. Understanding their capacity for brilliance helps them view themselves differently.

I can't find the words to describe how low my self-esteem was when I started out as an undergraduate student. I couldn't afford books, and for the first few months of school, I struggled academically. I was anxious and depressed and miserable.

Most of my fellow students didn't have to struggle so hard to succeed. Their parents paid for their tuition and books. After I graduated, I remember sitting in the auditorium and holding my degree. I looked around at the other graduates and thought, *I got the same damn degree you did, but I had to climb a hundred more mountains.*

I began to feel a bit indestructible, because while the other graduates learned that they could get degrees, I learned I could conquer mountains.

I want all my clients to feel that same way. Their psychological issues aren't what is important. Despite those issues, they've achieved remarkable things. Recognizing that opens minds. It empowers people. It creates lasting change. That is the point of therapy. Examining problems, on the other hand, can derail therapy.

Problems are everywhere, and therefore aren't relevant. For example, we can agree that there is no perfect person on the planet, meaning every person has some level of problem. If that's true, the pursuit of perfection is inherently flawed because we're never going to achieve it. And if that's true, the wiser course of action is to work toward becoming the very best version of ourselves *with* problems, instead of racking our brains on how to solve them.

Expending energy trying to do so is actually the root of depression and anxiety, because no matter how hard you work, when you look in the mirror, you're still going to see flaws.

Strangely, if you can fall in love with your flaws, then depression and anxiety can't exist. And one way to fall in love with them is to own them as part of your story.

I did just that. All of a sudden, I went from being totally ashamed of being poor—even to the extent of actively trying to hide it—to claiming it.

While my fellow graduates received the same degree as I did, with every privilege available to them, I had to claw my way through school because of my poverty. I borrowed books and studied from library copies. I once got a C on a test because my professor wanted me to read a fourth-edition book, and the only version available to me was the second edition in the library. Only 75 percent of the content overlapped, and I got 72 percent on the test. I came to realize that, given the circumstances, 72 percent was a really great score.

I started to recognize the hero in me, and I was determined to practice therapy in a way that made my clients feel just as heroic.

Now, I didn't know I was going to be writing books in the future. I had no idea I'd travel the world and meet someone like Adam. I just wanted to help people live better lives. I didn't even want credit for it. I just wanted to see people smile more.

I believe suffering is unnecessary, and I determined to make an impact on the amount of suffering people had to experience.

I didn't know the SFBT community would try to shun me for being so successful. I didn't know I'd have a million-dollar enterprise. At the time I was just a poor kid who thought suffering was inevitable. I even came close to killing myself. However, once I realized that suffering is unnecessary, I took it upon myself to let the whole world know. And the only approach that honored that way of thinking was solution focused brief therapy.

I believe in it 100 percent, and I have seen it work miracles with my clients.

Dig in deep as you read this book, start practicing SFBT, become proficient in it, and watch it work miracles with your clients too.

Chapter 3

He's the DJ,
I'm the Rapper

Friends before Colleagues

Diving Deep with Elliott

Back in 1988, the actor Will Smith, who was then known in the rap world as the Fresh Prince, released a second album with DJ Jazzy Jeff, who would later become his co-star on the television series *The Fresh Prince of Bel-Air*. The album was named after one of its songs, "He's the DJ, I'm the Rapper." Whenever people ask me to explain the pragmatics of how Adam and I work together, that's what I think of: "He's the DJ, I'm the rapper," only, "He's the researcher, I'm the clinician." Each role is important and complementary to the other.

Adam and I came into the world of solution focused brief therapy at relatively the same time. When we met, I was excited to find someone close to my age and developmental phase who was bold enough to go against the status quo. He wasn't afraid to critique and expand upon some of the traditional methods in our field because he understood, like I did, that part of growth and analysis involves critiquing.

I think Adam was also happy to have met someone who was good at practicing SFBT because, as a researcher, he loved watching therapy but found it hard to find clinicians who were not only good at their work but also willing to record their sessions. I was happy to share mine.

That's why I always say, "He's the DJ, I'm the rapper." There are two definitive jobs in our partnership: researching SFBT and practicing it.

There was also a personal connection between us. I just liked Adam. Part of our interactions involved work, and we totally nerded out over it. But I was also keenly aware that I'd just met a very special person. We laughed and had fun together. We didn't just talk about work; we talked about faith, life, and family.

Another reason why I compare us to DJ Jazzy Jeff and the Fresh Prince is because the DJ and the rapper were friends before they were artists. I'd say the same thing about us. Adam and I were friends before we were colleagues, and we will be friends through it all.

How We Met

A Closer Look with Adam

Elliott and I met in 2008 at a conference in Austin, Texas. We were introduced by a mutual colleague, said hello, and that was it. Fast-forward to two years later, and the three of us—Elliott, our colleague, and I—all happened to be going to the same three-day conference in Malmö, Sweden, where we would be the only American attendees.

When we arrived, we met up, and Elliott and I realized we still needed to pay the conference fee. They wouldn't take credit cards, though, so we had to walk to an exchange place to get Swedish money. We each needed 450 U.S. dollars, which converted to about 3,700 Swedish kronor. The exchange place gave both of us a thick stack of cash, and we kept joking that we felt so rich.

On the walk back to the hotel, Elliott started opening up to me. "This is the first time I'm speaking internationally," he said, "and when I looked at the program, I realized several well-known solution focused professionals are going to be speaking at the same time as I am. I don't think anyone's going to come to my workshop."

"Of course they will," I reassured him.

He glanced at his stack of kronor and smirked at me. "How about we make a bet? If more than ten people come to my workshop, I'll give you this nine thousand."

I laughed. "Deal."

That bet became our running joke. At the hotel, we paid our fees and split up when the conference began. I went to one workshop, and he went to another. Afterward, we both came out looking for our mutual friend. She was nowhere to be found, so we decided to go to the next workshop together. That kept happening throughout the day. We'd look for our friend, never find her, and continue to attend classes together.

At the end of the day, we went on a walk around Malmo to do a little sightseeing. We talked about things we liked or didn't like about what we'd been learning at the conference, and we realized we felt the same way about the solution focused approach—which happened to be very different from the way other therapists were practicing it.

"We should do a research study," I proposed. Elliott was hesitant at first—remember, he's the clinician, I'm the researcher—but I talked him into it. That got us excited, and we began to brainstorm other projects as well.

That walk together ended up being life-changing for us. Most importantly, it became very clear that our friendship should continue. Yes, we were on the same page about how we viewed SFBT, but beyond that we were laughing and having fun.

By the time we finished our walk, Elliott said, "I think we've just outlined thirty years' worth of work." Turns out it was much more than that. Eleven years later, neck-deep in all we do together, we realize we have decades of work yet to come. Nothing is more exciting.

For the record, Elliott lost that bet with me. Plenty of people showed up for his workshop; he definitely owed me that 3,700 kronor. He put off paying and we found ourselves at another conference, where he hedged a new bet: "How about I'll owe you double or nothing if no more than ten people come to my new workshop?"

Again, he lost. Since then, Elliott has bet me double or nothing so many times that he currently owes me 18 million American dollars. He's declared his "double or nothing" days are over.

Fine by me. I'll take my $18 million and run.

Tenacity, Belief, and Love

Diving Deep with Elliott

Adam helped me level up in my work because he's an unbelievably tenacious person and the most innovative researcher in our field. He pushed me to explain the things I did naturally as a clinician, which made me more attentive during my therapy sessions and, in turn, made me a much better teacher. He would never take "I don't know" for an answer. He'd say, "Go figure out the reason."

The foundation of SFBT is to believe in people, and I've always known that Adam believed in me. When he believes in someone, he's not capable of holding back his efforts to bring out the very best in that person. That's why he pushed me so hard through my "I don't knows." He was confident that if I didn't know the answer right away, I could eventually find it, and he wouldn't be doing me any justice if he stopped digging for it.

I'd often come back a week or so later and say, "Adam, you're really annoying, and I want to punch you in the face, but I now know the answer."

"Great," he'd reply. "Let's move on to my next question."

Those kinds of discussions went on for two years, before we ever wrote or published anything. I challenge you to find anyone in this field who has done the same. We did it because we enjoyed the conversation, we enjoyed the work, and above all we enjoyed the time spent together. He wanted me to realize my full potential, and I wanted him to realize his.

Solution focused brief therapy became the vehicle for our friendship, and in many ways, that's what this book is really about—friendship and love.

Adam and I decided long ago to use love as our tool, and we want the same for you. Love this work, love your clients, and love yourself. Understand that love is your power.

Our Synergy

A Closer Look with Adam

Anyone who has met Elliott knows he's a very passionate person. Without him in the mix, my research might become overly intellectual, but he brings the passion and humanness to what I do. To be honest, though, it was hard to capture that passion in research. How do people study "human"?

I tried to boil it down to its common denominators, and from there I had to figure out how to research and articulate it. We eventually called it the stance, which you'll read all about in the next section of the book.

Therapists are used to doing their work alone in a vacuum. Many of them get all the way through school without a live supervisor or a professor even watching their sessions. How therapists are evaluated is based on their own perception of their sessions. In research, that's a completely flawed information system.

The only way to get really good at therapy is to record it, watch it, and evaluate it. Before I even met Elliott, he was doing that—recording his sessions and watching them to get better. Beyond that, he was also willing to share his recordings with me. Most therapists are too scared to let other people see their work or they're too scared to put ideas into conversations with colleagues that aren't effective. Elliott has always been brave and humble in that regard.

We soon became accountability partners. We'd call each other once a week and talk for at least an hour. Leading up to those calls, he'd send me a DVD of his latest recorded sessions, and I'd watch them and take copious notes. Over the phone, I'd dig even further into his process.

Right from the beginning, there was a high level of excitement and trust between us, a mutual understanding of "I can tell you're doing your very best work, so I'm also going to do mine."

I'm sure we both would have been successful in our field without each other. We both would have been happy in our individual realms. But there's a synergy that comes when we're together. We're definitely better as a team.

We've taught as a pair countless times now, and we've learned to trust that our synergy will happen. It typically goes like this . . . Elliott speaks first—I call him the storyteller. He'll launch into a great story and tell it with his signature enthusiasm and passion. Always in sync, I know just when to step in and pick up the discussion. I usually focus on the teaching points he's brought up. Sometimes these teaching points aren't things Elliott mentioned overtly, but instead they're points embedded or implied in what he said. Often I find myself elaborating on subtle points that Elliott can take for granted because this is such a natural part of who he is and how he lives his life. From there, we tag-team our way through the rest of the presentation, consistently on the same page with each other.

Beyond our synergy, another defining aspect of our relationship is how we push one another outside of our comfort zones. He's constantly dragging me into things I probably never would have done or have chosen to do, especially when they involve speaking in front of people. And I'm constantly dragging him into things he probably never would have done or would have chosen to do, such as diving into complex and ambitious research projects.

In the end, we're both grateful. If Elliott pulls me into something, I trust it's going to get infinitely better because we're doing it together. With him, anything can be enjoyable.

Regardless of who dragged whom into any given situation, by the time we're done, we always end up saying, "That was great! I'm so glad we did that!"

Elliott's Story

Diving Deep with Elliott

The first memory I have of my father is of him bathing me gently and holding me up in front of a mirror while drying me off. I thought he was the most awesome dad in the world, and I wanted to be just like him.

On Saturday mornings, we ate breakfast at the same time. He'd sit down to eat a bowl of cereal, and he'd hold the bowl in his left hand and the spoon in his right. I tried to hold my own bowl similarly, but I struggled with my little two-and-a-half-year-old hands. It wasn't long before I dropped the bowl and spilled the cereal. As a punishment, my father spanked me aggressively, even though I was only a toddler.

These two events—being bathed lovingly and spanked roughly—happened in close proximity. It should come as no surprise then to learn that my life as a child was filled with lies, fear, and anxiety. It was also a life spent trying to please my father . . . or at the very least, trying not to upset him.

He was violent with everyone in my family—my two brothers, Mom, and me. I didn't feel like I could protect any of us from him, especially my mom. When I was 10 years old, my parents had a terrible fight, and my mother tried to defend herself by attempting to bite off his finger. He had to bandage it for a long time afterward because it was so gouged.

That event caused my self-esteem to decline even further, because I didn't know how to keep my mother safe from my father, even though on a logical level I knew that wasn't my responsibility.

Around that same time, when we were living in Boston after moving from Chicago, my father left my mother for the first time. Until then we had been a middle-class family, but afterward we became a very low-income family. My mother raised my brothers and me on only $17,000 a year. My dad came and went, but he was always around, especially on the weekends—which was when the violence continued to happen.

When I was 19 years old, my mom had a nervous breakdown that resulted in us moving to Texas to live closer to her sister and farther away from my father. In his physical absence, my life started to get better, but when he saw proof of that improvement during his infrequent visits, he'd overtly try to pull me down to feeling miserable again. I couldn't escape him.

When he was gone, he'd try to parent me over the phone, and his methods were aggressive, controlling, and outright mean. Despite that, I still sought his approval, and my life revolved around obtaining it.

Before we moved, I'd attended college at the University of Massachusetts–Dartmouth, but in Texas I had to restart my freshman year all over again. I felt horrible about myself. I had no money or resources. Not only was I starting over again, I was doing so in worse financial circumstances.

That was the darkest year of my life. I spent a majority of it not just contemplating but also accepting that I was going to commit suicide. Life as I knew it was not worth living, I told myself, so I wanted out.

I didn't feel sad. People often associate suicidality with sadness or even depression, but I believe it's associated with hopelessness, which was definitely the case for me.

Colleges are difficult places to be when you're poor and different. I'd watch my peers walk to the mailbox to get gifts from their families, be it food, clothes, a computer, or money. Meanwhile, I had nothing.

The best way I can describe how I felt is I had no hope that my father's abuse and its repercussions were ever going to stop. I could see them extending throughout the rest of my life.

If this is life, I thought, *I don't want one.*

Everybody else seemed to get a better one than me.

One day I was lying down in my dorm room, having fully accepted that as soon as I got the courage I was going to take my life.

It was then I had an epiphany: if I died, everyone was going to think something was wrong with me. My eulogy would be, "Elliott was sad. Elliott was depressed."

But that wasn't my issue—my father's abuse was the reason I'd been pushed to this point—and somehow I couldn't tolerate the thought of dying if that untruth would spread about me.

I wouldn't have minded if people said, "Elliott died because he got an unfair shake at life," but I didn't want them thinking I died because I had personal issues.

So there I was in my dorm room, when I realized that dying because of my father's problems was unacceptable. I couldn't do it. And if dying for his problems was unacceptable, then I needed to discover how to live for myself.

Immediately, I changed the way I lived my life. I started by setting boundaries with my father. I gave him three rules: he couldn't yell at me, he couldn't call me names, and he couldn't hit me. "If you can do those three things," I said, "I'm quite happy to have a relationship with you."

We never spoke again. He wasn't willing to follow my rules.

Even though that year was the hardest one of my life, it was also the most satisfying. It was the year I learned I could protect myself emotionally. It was the year I learned that if I could stand up to my dad, I could accomplish absolutely anything.

I became utterly fearless. I became more faithful and spiritual. Above all, I became a man who could slay a dragon. I took control of my life. I knew hard days might come again in the future, but I was empowered with the knowledge that I'd already defeated the biggest and scariest dragon. Every other dragon would never be as threatening.

That day in my dorm room I decided to go on an adventure, and it was an adventure of discovery. I knew what life had been like when I spent all of it trying to please my father. What I didn't know is what life could be like if I lived authentically as Elliott Connie.

My internal self-talk transformed. For the first time I began trying to achieve personal pride and satisfaction. I'd failed at trying to be who my dad wanted me to be, and I learned I could handle that failure. I might as well try to be who I was supposed to be.

And if I failed at that, so what? At least I'd fail while being true to myself. That new outlook was incredibly freeing.

The next semester, I worked out regularly and lost 50 pounds. I met my wife. I got a 4.0 GPA. I switched my major from marine biology to psychology because I was interested in the brain. I knew my father would say, "You can't make any money in psychology. What are you going to do with that degree?" But I didn't care. I started making decisions on the basis of what felt right to me, and on that basis alone.

I no longer think about challenges in terms of being challenges. I don't consider quitting or failing, because I know I can endure anything. I'm used to reaching milestones that should have been simple but instead were very difficult. Because of that, difficulty doesn't make any difference to me.

I've developed a "roger that" mentality. If I have to race someone around the block, and the other person gets a bike while I have to run, I say, "Roger that." I don't care what advantage anyone else has. My philosophy is that if I've got to do life hard, I'll do it hard. And when I accomplish what I set out to achieve, I want people to know that I didn't ask for any favors. Despite the obstacles in my path, I crossed the finish line and won.

Looking back on the early years of my life, I'm grateful for the pain and suffering I had to live with because it made me a good psychotherapist. I empathize with my clients. I practice an approach that enables change without causing further suffering.

One of the hallmarks of solution focused brief therapy is that change doesn't have to take forever. I know because I lived it. When therapists rattle off statistics like, "It takes eighteen sessions to create lasting change," I say, "No, it doesn't." In a dorm room, in just a moment, I changed my life.

Change can happen instantaneously.

Adam's Story

A Closer Look with Adam

My view of people and what they're capable of comes from my own experience of having to be strong during difficult circumstances, as well as witnessing the people close to me face significant challenges with great capability.

I'm the fourth of five children, and when I was very young, my mom went back to work full-time. She worked the night shift at the hospital, and she would put us kids to bed, go to work, and be back home before we woke up. We never felt the impact of her being gone, though it took a toll on her. For seven years, she worked throughout the night, getting very little sleep and pushing her body to the limit.

When I was seven years old, I woke up one morning and my mother wasn't home. My dad told me she was still at the hospital. She'd had a heart attack and needed open-heart surgery, he said. She was going to have to stay in the hospital for two weeks while she began her recovery.

That was a life-changing experience for our family, and I came to appreciate my mother in a new light as I watched her regain her health and energy. She learned to pace herself better, though she never surrendered her desire to continue accomplishing incredible things.

A few years later, when I was in middle school, my mother and father decided to go back to school to receive their doctorate degrees. Not only would they be working full-time and going to school full-time, but my dad would also be serving as our church's stake president, a voluntary position in charge of overseeing several congregations across a large geographical area. Needless to say, my parents were very busy.

Many days would pass in which I wouldn't see them. My older sisters had grown into adults by this time and had moved out of the house, so my teenage brothers and I were the only ones at home.

I'm sure my parents couldn't tell you much about what happened during those years of my life. While I never viewed them as neglectful—they still provided for our needs and came to our school events—we were basically given free rein to govern ourselves. I had to learn very quickly how to become self-sufficient.

When I was 19 years old, I went on a church mission to England. I was given a calling to learn British Sign Language and work with Deaf people. In doing so, I watched how the Deaf community dealt with oppression and the pressure to assimilate from the hearing community, and how they rose up to advocate for their own culture, equal opportunity, and fair representation.

Again, I witnessed the remarkable capability that people have in overcoming adversity. This became more evident than ever after I married my wife, Becca, in 2002.

Both of us wanted to start a family, but that turned out to be very difficult because she had horrible pregnancies with severe morning sickness. She was put on bed rest often and vomited five to six times a day on average. She suffered miscarriages too. Bringing children into this world was extremely taxing on her.

After she gave birth to our first child, I said, "If we never do this again, I totally understand." But she wanted more children, even though each pregnancy became progressively worse. I kept telling her the same thing, "If we never do this again, I totally understand."

The only reason we have three children now is because Becca fought so hard for them.

Later in our marriage, in May 2019, she was diagnosed with breast cancer. Our youngest child was eight at the time—the same age I had been when my mom had her heart attack. History seemed to be repeating itself.

Over the span of three months, Becca had surgery and four rounds of chemo. That was followed by six weeks of daily radiation treatments. She lost all her hair, dealt with excruciating pain (worse than her pregnancies), and struggled because she couldn't take care of her family—the thing she loves most about life.

In December 2019, she finished her treatments, but her cancer-related trials weren't yet over. In March 2020 (when the nationwide emergency was declared), COVID-19 hit our world. As a household, we had to completely lock down. Our kids didn't go to in-person school, even when schools reopened in our area. Becca's doctors explained that for a year following her cancer treatments she would be immunocompromised. We had to implement strict measures to prevent her from catching the coronavirus.

After nearly a year of isolation due to cancer and another year of isolation due to COVID-19, Becca has come out stronger and better. On the day she was diagnosed with cancer, I asked her how she knew she would be able to handle all this. She thought for a minute, cried for a few more, and then answered, "Because, I can do hard things!" This became our mantra.

Recently, I asked Becca what life is like nearly two years after completing her treatments. She said she would never want to go through that again, but she is so grateful for the lessons she learned, and the person she became as a result of these hard things. She mentioned that she appreciates the small things now, like being able to go to our kids' swim meets, going to the grocery store, and having the energy to stand up from a crouched position without feeling like she is going to fall over.

She also mentioned that even though her cancer and its repercussions were hard on our family, she is glad to know that we stand together and support each other. Now she has one more "hard thing" that she knows she can do.

As a husband, there is nothing worse than watching the person you love suffer so much, knowing there is nothing you can do to relieve the pain. Watching Becca push through challenge after challenge made me realize that she was proving not only to herself but also to me that she was stronger than we knew. Additionally, I realized that when we are the onlookers of other people in the midst of struggle, we are actually witnessing greatness. As people push through their hardest days, they manifest their greatest strength. Becca changed the way I see her, but more importantly, she has changed the way I see all people.

Elliott was also greatly touched by how Becca faced the challenge of cancer. He got a tattoo on his right wrist that says, "I can do hard things," written in Becca's handwriting. He is constantly trying to get me to get a tattoo as well, but so far he'll just have to be satisfied with Becca's mantra in her handwriting.

Elliott has been there for me in both the good times and the hard. For over a decade now, I've had the privilege of being his best friend and business partner, and I've tried my best to support him as well.

The racism he's endured as a Black therapist in a White-dominated field has been staggering and horrifying. There were times he called me, having decided he was going to leave the field because of the mistreatment he received. However, each time we would talk about the bigger mission that he has and we have together, and each time I committed to walk by his side again.

I am constantly amazed at his determination to teach people and to see the best in others, even when he isn't afforded that same courtesy. As with Becca's situation, I am often the onlooker while Elliott is the recipient of discrimination and oppression. But after 11 years, he just keeps getting more brilliant at his clinical work, his teaching and training, and living a generous life. It is an honor to watch his fortitude and ability "to do hard things"!

Where Elliott's adversity came firsthand, in many ways I was more of an observer of adversity. Perhaps my hardship in doing so wasn't as challenging as what my loved ones had to endure, but learning to remain hopeful during those difficulties has shaped who I've become, as well as increased my desire to research how meaningful conversation can access the greatness that is within the human soul.

While Elliott and I have confronted adversity from different angles, we've both reached the same outcome in our business and relationship—a united front committed to giving our very best in order to help people live happier and more purposeful lives.

Fighting Racism as Brothers:
The Moment We Became Something More

Diving Deep with Elliott

As a Black man in this field, I've experienced racism, exclusion, and discrimination—everything that goes along with being an overt minority. Adam, on the other hand, was in what we referred to as "the club," meaning he was on elite boards and in contact with influential professionals, many of whom were actively oppressing me, though I didn't think at the time that he realized that.

Over time, he started losing access to the club. People began to exclude him from projects and started distancing themselves. Secretly, I felt bad because I knew the reason had to do with my working relationship with him, and I didn't know if he was aware of it. As bright as he is, Adam is very . . . well, White. Would he be able to puzzle together what was happening and why? Prejudice wasn't something he'd had to endure on a daily basis, while it was a reality I'd been living with my whole life.

Eventually Adam began to remove his own access to the club. He resigned from organizations and severed relationships. It took me years to conjure up the strength to finally say to him, "I think the reason that ugly things are happening to you is because of your association with me."

Without missing a beat, he replied, "I know."

"You do?" I asked, taken aback.

He explained that when he'd decided to work with me years ago, he knew what it would cost him. He even had a conversation with his wife about it—there are no secrets between them. "With my eyes wide-open," Adam told me, "I decided to go down this path with you. And I don't regret it."

When I heard that, I broke down into tears. Until then, I didn't realize the extent of how much he believed in me and how much he'd willingly given up in order to work together. It struck me that our relationship was more than a partnership of colleagues who happened to be friends. We were different. This was commitment. This was unequivocal loyalty.

In an earlier chapter of the book, I mentioned how Adam and I had the opportunity to meet with Hezekiah Watkins, one of the Freedom Riders from the civil rights movement. During our conversation, we asked what he thought of a Black man like me and a White man like Adam partnering together in the present day, given everything he had been through in 1961.

Hezekiah replied by telling us the story of how he'd been shot at when he was fighting for justice. "As I ran from the shooter," he said, "I looked to my left and saw a White guy running beside me. 'That's my brother,' I realized. His race didn't matter because we were both running from bullets while trying to create change."

I felt the same way when Adam said he knew what he was doing when he first embarked on this journey with me. He became more than an associate in that moment, more than a friend. He became my brother. He was willing to be shot at beside me—and he has been—fully aware of the consequences. Knowing he did it on purpose is the most touching thing I will ever experience.

Adam and I often say to each other, "I didn't know we could become any closer," and then something happens, and we inevitably do become closer. This was one of those moments. Our relationship became something more than it had been—and that something more has continued to grow ever since.

Adam is often mistaken for weak because he's small in stature and often soft-spoken. But he's the single strongest person I know. When people attempt to bully him, I sit back, pop some popcorn, and think, *Wow, this is going to be fun*. The man can't be intimidated.

He once resigned from a board that took issue with our project for racist reasons, and they had an exit meeting to try to pressure him to stay on their research committee. He was on that call for two hours, and if you know Adam, that call could have lasted for two years and he still wouldn't have backed down. When he believes he's in the right, he will not shrink. It's just not part of his character.

"I don't know how it happened," I say when people ask how he and I became what we are now. The only answer that seems to scratch the surface is, "God touched it."

While I don't know how it happened, I did recognize *when* it was happening—and that was the moment I found out he was willing to run from bullets with me.

In order for Adam to support me, I've had to authentically show him who I am. And in order for me to support him, he's had to authentically show me who he is. That has allowed us then to simultaneously show the world who we are . . . and when doing that becomes hard, we're there for each other.

No matter what, I know Adam is at my side, saying, "All right, I've got you. Now go be you. When the bullets start flying, I'll be right here beside you."

Pursuing the Outcome Despite Adversity

A Closer Look with Adam

Adversity is one of the most important elements of our combined story. Even in a field where therapists are supposed to promote viewing others as wonderful, Elliott has been treated horribly because of his race.

Several years ago I was on the research committee for a national association that reported to a board. The committee asked me to spearhead a project, and I asked if Elliott could help. He wasn't on the committee, but he was perfect for the job. The committee agreed, and Elliott and I put together a proposal that we sent to the board for approval.

The board sent back a long list of stipulations. Among other things, we were told we couldn't put our names on the project or use it to promote our business—neither of which we'd planned on anyway. We would be doing the project on behalf of the research committee and giving them the credit, a fact the board would have well known, especially since the president was also a member of the research committee. She knew firsthand how this project came about, and that Elliott and I had no intention of doing it for our own personal gain.

It became clear what the board's stipulations were really regarding.

I submitted a three-page statement, addressing each of their stipulations. I was frank in saying how I doubted that any of their concerns would have arisen if I'd been doing the project with anyone else. "I can't help but wonder," I added, "why are you targeting Elliott in this way?"

For his own part, Elliott submitted a two-page statement that detailed multiple instances in which the board had treated him unfairly. "Does this have something to do with my race?" he wrote. "And if it doesn't, what does it have to do with?"

In essence, we both told them, "Your actions seem very racist."

We submitted a five-page response in total, and in reply, the board only wrote back five sentences that fundamentally said, "If we hurt your feelings, we didn't mean to."

That was the end of the rope for me. I wanted nothing more to do with them. I dropped the project, resigned from the committee, and told Elliott, "We are no longer associating with any of these people."

Four years went by, and we never said anything about it publicly. The board never said a word about it either. All was quiet until Elliott made an unrelated comment on a public international forum.

Our field is very White-dominated, traditional, academic, and formal. Where other industries and professions are becoming more intolerant to racism, psychotherapy is still decades behind. Consequently, it needs to be "woke," for lack of a better term. Someone needed to call out what was happening in order for things to improve, and that someone was Elliott.

Coming from a formal culture myself, I've had to become accustomed to how bold Elliott is when he calls out racism. He has to manage these situations differently than I do as a White man. His example has inspired me, and I'm learning to confront racism more overtly and courageously.

In the comment Elliott made, he called out the board for their racism toward him four years ago. Someone who had been on that board replied by writing an account of what he claimed had happened, but it was significantly flawed and erroneous.

I wasn't on the forum, but the account was slanderous enough that people started reaching out to ask if I'd seen it. I joined the forum to do so, and once I did, I couldn't remain silent. I responded to the board member, and what I wrote was so lengthy that it filled two entries. I listed every false point he made and corrected them with information taken verbatim from our past e-mail exchange.

Several years have now passed from the time of that initial racist encounter, and members of the board still treat Elliott poorly. In a likewise manner, a continuous stream of people in our field have also tried to hold him back or discredit him.

In spite of the many roadblocks that have stood in the way of Elliott being successful, he reacts like he always does—by just continuing to pursue his desired outcome.

That's the focus of solution focused brief therapy—pursuing your outcome in the face of adversity. Elliott believes in this process so much that he never falters from his attitude of "I'll just keep going. I'll do my best."

Racist interactions aimed at him have been plain ridiculous at times. Once he was part of a Zoom call with the board of a different organization—ironically, one he and I started—and at a later date, one of the members accused him of saying something offensive during that session. To prove otherwise, Elliott offered to show her the Zoom recording, to which she replied, "Well, I know you didn't say it, but I think it's something you *would* say."

At another time, after I first started working with Elliott, a colleague we used to be close with approached me at a conference. "You need to be very careful whom you associate with," she said. "People are starting to assume that you're like Elliott."

I looked her in the face and replied, "I'm very aware of whom I'm associating with. And given this conversation, I think I've chosen correctly."

Time after time, as Elliott has faced blatant racism, he and I have had to adapt and keep pushing forward. It wasn't until we grew this big organization on our own—The Solution Focused Universe—that the profession came to view him as credible. Now he's a dominant force in our field, and all the people who oppressed him years ago are trying to get back in his good graces.

In many ways, Elliott's story of resilience reminds me of Insoo Kim Berg's. As we mentioned in a previous chapter, she traveled on foot hundreds of miles during the Korean War to deliver her brothers and herself to safety. Later in life, she developed a psychotherapy model based on perseverance despite obstacles, based on looking toward where you're going rather than where you've come from.

Elliott picked up that baton and expanded on Insoo's approach. He practices what he's lived and continues to live. He teaches about the power of change in a new way. And he's made that change for himself. He's built a seven-figure business from the ground up, undeterred by the people who have tried to tear him down. He finds hope in the darkest of circumstances.

While I compare Elliott to Insoo, I find that I relate to her husband, Steve de Shazer. Steve was very much the philosopher, the thinker, and the theorizer of the partnership, and Insoo was very much the clinician. Steve used to frequently say that he learned what solution focused brief therapy is all about by watching and analyzing Insoo as she practiced it.

I would say the same. I know everything I've learned about SFBT from watching Elliott practice it—he's brilliant at it. I've analyzed it and researched it and continued to be amazed by his gift at it.

Elliott calls us the DJ and the rapper, but he also compares us to Batman and Robin. "Sometimes I'm Batman and you're Robin," he says. "And sometimes I'm Robin and you're Batman." We're both okay with either role. We're fine to let the other person shine.

His strengths are different from mine, and mine are different from his. Both are important. Both are valuable. We completely respect that.

Our combined story has led us to trust one another implicitly. We've become stronger because so many people have tried to pull us apart.

I stand by what I told Elliott years ago, "With my eyes wide-open, I decided to go down this path with you. And I don't regret it."

PART II

The Stance

Chapter 4

ADOPT the Diamond Stance

Adopt a New Way of Thinking

Traditional psychotherapy is based on people's problems. Clinicians and psychiatrists are taught to use the *Diagnostic and Statistical Manual of Mental Disorders* (American Psychiatric Association, 2013), a handbook thicker than a phone book that categorizes all known mental health disorders. We're taught to first diagnose, then pick a therapy approach designed to fix that mental illness.

This problem-oriented lens in the field of psychotherapy is also reflected in the social constructs of our day. The news focuses on horrible events over uplifting ones. Medical doctors ask patients, "What's wrong?" instead of "What's going well?"

The tendency to want to fix problems is one of the main reasons clinicians choose psychotherapy as a career. "I was always the person people confided in," they say. "I gave good advice." Consequently, what they bring to the table in their practice is "I give good advice."

Our SFBT approach directly confronts that. As an SFBT therapist, your job is no longer to give advice. Your job is to co-construct your client's desired outcome, to ask questions, and to obtain a detailed description of the transformation your client is seeking.

This is difficult for therapists to hear because they're fixers. They believe problems are important, thanks to that narrative from society. They got into this field because they want to be saviors, but that's a slippery slope. Ego gets in the way when you're driven by the need to figure out what's wrong with another person.

In our approach, we overtly say there is no need to diagnose your clients. That tactic doesn't produce change. Although the symptoms of the various disorders may be present (and, therefore, a diagnosis may be relevant), treatment from an SFBT perspective is not contingent upon understanding the presence of the symptoms or relevant diagnosis. The stance along with the SFBT diamond model produces change. Without the stance, the method is bloodless. But in order to adopt the stance, you have to be willing to unlearn what you have been taught about psychotherapy, what you believe your role is, and what society has programmed you to believe is important in life.

This work isn't transformative only for clients, but also transformative for you. When you view your clients as capable and strong, it changes you—and how you do your job. Your perceptions directly impact your actions.

Let's say you're driving a car and somebody cuts you off. You can either view the other driver as a jerk, in which case you might honk at him, flip him off, or tailgate him. Or you can view him as someone who may be in a crisis, in which case you're more likely to have a kinder response. You might pull back, let him into your lane easier, or even wave at him.

At the end of the day, you only have control over your own part of an interaction with someone else. The same thing can be said of your role as a therapist.

Before a client even walks into your office, if you take the stance of viewing that person as great and competent, you also come to the therapy as a changed and better person. That version of you—the best you—will evoke the best in your client.

Recognize How You Show Up

A stance is a lens, a way of seeing people that shouldn't be confined to your work as a therapist. A stance isn't something to flip on and off like a light switch. It should remain on at all times—inside and outside of the therapy room. It should be consistent in your life. The stance we advocate that should come with you, from your everyday life, into the therapy room is one of being awe-inspired. We believe that you should live life in such a way that you are in awe of each person you meet. Awe should be the filter through which each interaction should be processed. Awe might cause you to be astonished or surprised. Perhaps you see a small child who is outstanding at playing a musical instrument. This talent should surprise you, in the best of ways, but you should be on the lookout for opportunities to be surprised—perhaps even asking children you encounter what special skills or talents they have, so they can surprise you. At other times awe will take the form of amazement or wonder. This amazement might occur when you hear from someone that, despite having a physical disability, they have risen to the top within a sporting event or they have tackled a physical adventure that many nondisabled individuals would never dream of attempting. We can be amazed by their ability to overcome hardship, but again, we should actively engage with people to be awestruck by them. We should hold a stance of awe, and we should engage with people from a place of awe within each interaction.

Think about religion. It becomes a filter for those who practice it. Everything you do or think runs through it. The stance we ask you to take in practicing solution focused brief therapy should also be a filter for your thoughts and actions. We want you to see greatness in others, then act on that greatness. The stance influences your own behavior.

To put it simply, a stance is how you show up in any given interaction. And therapists are often unaware of how they show up.

Let's say Adam arrives in a suit and tie to do in-home therapy visits with teens on the South Side of Chicago. When none of those kids open up to him, his takeaway might be that teens on the South Side of Chicago don't like therapy. Instead, perhaps those kids just don't like therapy in their homes from White men wearing suits and ties.

Be aware of how you show up. You play a role in how productive therapy is. It doesn't all fall on the client.

We often get e-mails from therapists asking, "What do you do with traumatized clients who can no longer see hope?" or "How do you handle clients who are incapable of answering questions other than saying, 'I don't know'?"

Our response is always the same. First of all, we don't view clients as incapable. For that matter, we don't believe people are incapable. Furthermore, we recognize our need to step up when our clients answer, "I don't know." We ask them better questions because we're aware that we contribute to the interaction.

Therapists often struggle to see how they contribute to difficulty. In over 15 years of teaching SFBT, we've never once heard a therapist say, "I think that session didn't go well because I'm not any good at this, and I want to get better." Instead, they blame their clients.

"He isn't ready for change."

"She waited too long to come to therapy."

"He's resistant."

"She doesn't know how to answer my questions."

Therapists never say, "You know, maybe I need to improve myself."

Interestingly, in other areas of life, people admit their shortcomings. If Elliott tried to bake macarons and burned them, he would say, "I need to become a better baker."

"Resistant clients" are actually just clients trying to protect themselves. How can they be vulnerable with someone whom they believe can't understand them? How can they open up when they feel as though they're at a disadvantage?

When you walk into your office, you take on a tremendous amount of privilege—simply because the client is sitting in your space. In our approach to SFBT, we ask you to do everything you can to minimize that imbalance of power.

Let go of social constructions that cause more inequality. Beware of clinging to the stance that your role as a therapist is to give good advice. By doing so, you inadvertently exacerbate your position of privilege. Meanwhile, your clients sense their loss of power and disengage. They believe you don't care, you don't see their potential, and furthermore, you're not interested in changing your viewpoint. Take the first step to equality by acknowledging your privilege, especially when it's difficult.

Be Willing to Give Up Power

In order to practice effective solution focused brief therapy, you must be willing to give up power, and that's tough for most therapists. They enjoy being the voice of authority.

Reluctance to give up power also shows up when therapists say, "I don't work with X population." They may as well be saying, "I don't feel powerful when I work with X population."

If X = teenagers, what they mean is, "I don't feel powerful when I work with teenagers, because teenagers are really good at taking power."

If you're not willing to share power with your clients, the result is feeling incompetent in your work. The easy response is to say, "I'm out. I don't work with teenagers."

Our stance is to abolish these self-imposed limitations. View yourself as capable of greatness with any population. Your greatness comes from being willing to allow others to show their own greatness.

Did you know the two most common populations that therapists refuse to work with are domestic abusers and child molesters? Why? Therapists sum up those people based on only one type of action, and they don't want any part of it. That's completely counter to the stance of recognizing that your clients may have made grievous mistakes but also asking yourself, "What other version of them do I need to talk to in order to inspire change?" Only that version has the power to quit making those mistakes.

Stop looking at people as if they're only one thing. Just as you remove limitations you place on yourself, remove limitations you place on others. Work with the best version of your clients so they understand that they have power in your office—power to contribute to therapy and power to do something about *why* they are there.

If your client has a terrible addiction, the only person who can change that is your client. This is why we struggle with the idea that the therapist is the fixer. The *client* is the fixer. Clients are the ones who have to achieve their desired outcomes.

Suggestions for Giving Up Power

◆ First and foremost, acknowledge that simply by sitting in the chair of the clinician, you have more power in the relationship than the client.

◆ Don't give your client advice. Remember that they are the expert of their own social location and they have a better idea about what will work for them than you do.

◆ Only talk about what the client invites you to talk about. You should use their exact language whenever possible.

◆ Avoid using stereotypical ideas and language such as, "As an African American, how do you experience . . ." or "As a lesbian, have you ever had someone . . ." Although these questions may come from good intentions, they force the client to focus on experiences that may be irrelevant to their best hopes.

◆ Remember, your job is just to get a description of the client's best hopes!

Give the Client the Reward

Diving Deep with Elliott

Long before I learned about solution focused brief therapy, I had a job doing in-home family therapy in a program driven by cognitive behavioral therapy. I worked with teens, and the program identified them as drug users.

One day my supervisor said my client Caden (name changed), had just received the results of his fourth consecutive clean drug test. "Good job, Elliott," they told me.

I had a knee-jerk reaction to their compliment. Why were they giving me credit? I didn't stop using drugs. Caden did. They didn't give him any praise, however. Instead, they expressed doubts. "Caden, we're concerned you won't be able to keep this up."

As you can imagine, that did nothing to further his confidence.

You can be the greatest therapist in the world, but your client is the person who has to go into that world and say, "No more drugs." That requires the building up of your client. There's no place for any tearing down. Your client has to leave each therapy session feeling more powerful than when they entered it.

I'm not talking about empowerment, which implies that your client's power source is from you. I'm talking about your client's *inherent* power and your role to help them see it. With that power, they can stop using drugs or make whatever changes they desire.

Beware of the tendency to communicate doubt. Therapists do it all the time. Human beings do it all the time. Doubt is damaging, and doubt perpetuates doubt. People are impressionable, and doubt impacts them for the worse.

Imagine a teen girl saying to her parents, "I'm going to try to win at the swim meet today." What if her parents were to respond, "Hmm, I don't know if you should try to win"? That doubt would transfer to the girl. It would impact her negatively.

In another scenario, let's say a man tells his therapist, "I want to get clean from drugs." What if the therapist replied, "Well, you're going to have to take it slowly and start with something more manageable"? That therapist has just communicated that getting clean is beyond his client's capability. Even if that were true (which it never is), how would that help the client?

For the record, we can give countless examples of people who became clean remarkably fast by using SFBT.

Therapists also have a tendency to project their own limitations onto their clients. When you place yourself in your clients' shoes, be careful not to bring your own baggage. If you believe you'd have difficulty getting clean, your instinct is to assume they will also struggle in the same way.

Thoughts That Indicate You Are Projecting Your Own Ideas about Limitations

♦ Believing the client when they answer with "I don't know" and moving on to a different question

♦ Thinking that clients with "significant" presenting complaints/problems may not be suitable for SFBT without even having a conversation with them

♦ Thinking that the "best-hopes" question may not be the right place to start because "this client is in such a difficult situation that they aren't in a place that they can begin to think about being hopeful"

♦ Feeling stuck because the client asks something like, "Why are you asking me these strange questions?"

♦ Thinking that you have some good advice or insight that the client needs in order to feel better

♦ Believing that psychoeducation is the best way forward

People have different strengths. It isn't your role to place limitations on what others can achieve. Whether your clients accomplish what they desire or not, working toward that outcome will make them better people. They'll develop skills and discipline they wouldn't have obtained otherwise.

What matters is they're going to become who they want to be on the journey. Maybe along the way they decide, "Actually, I'm going to use these new skills to go in a different direction."

That's fine. It's the *becoming* that's important.

A changed person can accomplish wonders.

Think of how you've surprised yourself in your own life. I bet you've achieved things you never thought were possible. I bet you never imagined you'd be X. But one day you woke up and you were X.

Draw from your own experiences of hope. Remember how you became something new, something wonderful. View your clients with that same lens of remarkable capability.

When you see the superhero in yourself, you'll see the super-hero in others. You can't view in another person what you can't view in yourself. That's the essence of the stance. Once you understand your own ability and amazingness, you'll develop the lens to see others as if they have all the potential in the world.

The Stance of Radical Acceptance

A Closer Look with Adam

Human beings spend a lot of energy trying to figure out how to overcome differences with each other. But Elliott and I believe overcoming differences isn't what's important. *Accepting* differences is. He totally accepts me. I totally accept him. And because we've done that from the beginning, our work relationship shifted and became more personal.

He makes fun of me and says I have no swagger, but he never asks me to change the way I dress. He never asks me to change anything about myself. He just says, "That's exactly who you are, and it's okay. I like you because of that."

We believe solution focused therapists should also take this same stance of radical acceptance with their clients—even those who are child abusers or part of another written-off population. Radically accept they are phenomenal. Take the time to understand how that's possible.

Child abusers usually engage in destructive behavior because they feel out of control and belittled. To cope, they take power from children to stabilize their own feelings. Once they recognize they already have an infinite amount of power within themselves, then taking power from small kids suddenly seems meaningless. SFBT helps them identify that power.

To practice effective SFBT you need to cultivate a solid relationship with your clients. If you belittle or doubt them, you damage that relationship. It's essential to convey that you trust them. You have their best interests at heart. Without that understanding, why would they trust you in return? How could they be fully vulnerable during therapy? It wouldn't be safe.

Do all you can to foster the therapist–client relationship. Convey complete and utter acceptance in your clients. Whoever they are, accept them and treat them as deserving people.

Fostering the SFBT Therapist–Client Relationship

♦ Listen with a caring ear. Hear only the best about the person.

♦ Convey warmth and acceptance of each client answer.

♦ Use the client's exact language whenever possible.

♦ Only talk about the client's desired outcome.

♦ Honor the problem (don't ignore it or minimize it), but focus on the parallel experience of strength and resilience.

♦ Communicate through loving language that you believe completely in the client and their abilities.

ADOPT the Stance

In order to master the diamond—the framework of SFBT strategies and techniques designed to guide you through each session of therapy—you must first ADOPT the stance. The five components of the stance are:

- A is for autonomy: Autonomy is sacred.
- D is for difference: SFBT is a difference-led approach.
- O is for outcome: SFBT is an outcome-led approach.
- P is for presuppose: Presuppose the best in your client.
- T is for trust: Trust your client's capability.

In the next few chapters, we'll discuss these five components in detail. Adopt the stance—truly accept it and put it into practice—and you'll realize your full potential as an exceptional SFBT therapist.

Chapter 5

Autonomy Is Sacred

The Moment I Let Go
of Fixing My Clients

Diving Deep with Elliott

Early in my career, parents would often come to me and say, "My child is off the path. Can you fix them?" Couples I worked with often had this same plea. They wanted me to fix their relationship—usually by fixing the other person.

These requests always placed a tremendous amount of pressure on me because I had no control over another person's behavior. I never will. How was I supposed to fix someone? Was that part of my job in helping people?

I did my best to give advice, homework, and compliments to my clients, as I had been taught to do as a psychotherapist, until the time I worked with a married couple who completely changed my approach.

When they came to me for help, I was a super green therapist, having just received my master's degree the previous year. During our first session together, the husband and wife were at each other's throats. I tried to think of suggestions I could give them, but for the first time in my therapy career, I refrained from giving advice, simply because I didn't know how to do that in this situation. It was so intense I couldn't figure out what I should or shouldn't say.

For context, the wife had reconnected with a man from her past on Myspace, which her husband referred to as "Divorce Space." The husband wanted his wife to share her Internet passwords with him, but she refused.

"I didn't do anything with the other man," she told her husband. "Yes, we planned to meet up, but nothing happened. Meanwhile, you have ignored me for years. If you wanted me, you should have shown you wanted me this whole time. You have no right to ask for my passwords."

I don't remember how well or how poorly I conducted this session. All I clearly recall is not giving the couple advice.

A few days later, they came back to therapy, and everything between them seemed fine. They were acting like a completely different couple.

"What's changed?" I asked, perplexed.

The husband smiled at his wife. "She gave me her passwords, and now I feel perfectly secure in our relationship."

Amazed, I asked her, "What changed to allow you to give him your passwords?"

She affectionately placed her hand on her husband's leg. "He made the bed with me in it."

I wasn't sure if I'd heard her correctly. "What do you mean?"

She grinned coyly. "Have you ever had the feeling of fresh sheets dropped on you?"

I was beginning to understand. "Like when your parents tuck you in as a child?"

She nodded. "When we woke up one morning this past week, my husband picked up the sheets and dropped them on me as I was lying in bed. Then he did it again. He did it three times, and afterward I knew he cared about me. I wanted him to feel secure, so I gave him my passwords. Everything has been fine since."

I stared at both of them, astonished. No matter how hard I had tried during our first session, I could never in a million years have thought of giving the husband the advice to go home and make the bed with his wife in it.

Perhaps therapy wasn't about me solving the problem, I realized. Perhaps therapy was about me evoking the best in people so they could solve their own problems.

My aim from that time forward was to figure out how to structure sessions in a way that honored the autonomy of my clients. With that in place, they could claim their own power to make life-changing improvements.

The Importance of Autonomy and Agency

The traditional definition of *autonomy* is the right to govern oneself. We fully believe in that right. As a therapist, if you step over that line and assign your clients a task or try to problem-solve, you've limited their ability to govern themselves.

When you begin a session by asking your client, "What are your best hopes?" you're essentially asking, "How do you want to govern yourself?"

In other words, you're saying, "Tell me what you want to do here" or "Tell me what you want to talk about." The rest of the session is structured around your client's answer.

If you honor your client's ability to govern herself throughout the entire session and then get to the end and take that away by dictating what she should do from that point, you've undone what you've spent the whole session building.

Another word that goes in conjunction with *autonomy* is *agency*, which means the right to choose. If you step in and remove your client's ability to choose, you're not letting them live up to their full potential.

If you were to assign a task or homework, oftentimes your client will go home and do exactly what you've requested, but that limits what she could have done.

The previous story is the perfect example of this. If Elliott had said to the wife, "Go home and have a conversation about what it would take for you to share your passwords with your husband," she probably would have gone home and had that conversation, but it would have limited other possible courses of action. Perhaps the husband would have never made the bed with her in it, which ended up being the catalyst for improving their marriage.

When you trust that your clients can govern themselves, you let them choose their own paths, whatever those happen to be—even if the consequence is them not benefitting from therapy.

Therapists often say they want to empower their clients, but what they actually do is merely encourage their clients. Empowerment conveys something bolder. It means giving clients the free choice—the agency to do what they want with a session. Failure is one of those choices.

Your clients can choose to meet with you and not do anything differently in their lives. Or they can choose to meet with you and never be the same human being again.

Most therapists don't honor their clients' choices and therefore spend a lot of time and energy encouraging change—a limited and exhausting approach that leads to burnout. Instead, when agency is honored, clients take responsibility for their actions, whether good or bad. They don't give you credit for their success or blame you for their failure. They own the outcome, and they're much more likely to make choices that are congruent to the lives they want to lead.

That's the brilliant thing about human beings. When you give them a choice, they will most often choose what's good for them.

The Balance of Co-Construction

In regard to solution focused brief therapy, co-construction is the maximum collaboration of client agency, which is expressed through the client's language, along with the expertise of the clinician to structure a therapy session around the client's desired outcome. You know you are co-constructing effectively when you are picking up the client's exact words and building your next question with those words intact. This co-construction is at peak effectiveness when the client's exact words are being used to create a detailed description about the presence of their desired outcome. You can co-construct anything, but in SFBT we co-construct desired-outcome descriptions.

Effective co-construction in the way that we advocate requires hard work, courage, and discipline. There's no room for laziness or cowardice.

Giving your client agency doesn't mean he should lead the conversation, however. Some therapists take the position that if a client randomly brings up Corn Flakes, they need to talk about Corn Flakes. Instead, it's your job to keep the conversation on track and relevant to the client's pursuit of achieving his desired outcome.

Elliott once worked with a client who was addicted to crystal meth. Elliott asked him, "What's the first thing you would do on a day in which you woke up and didn't use crystal meth?"

"I'd be thinking about something different," the client answered.

"What would that be?" Elliott asked.

"Cake," he replied.

It was Elliott's job then to connect cake with sobriety. As a therapist, that was his whole purpose of being there. The client didn't really want to talk about cake; he wanted to talk about cake as it related to being sober. That's where Elliott had to bring his expertise.

Some therapists believe solution focused brief therapy is a nonexpert stance, but that isn't true. You may not be an expert on the client, but you're absolutely an expert on the process. Part of that means keeping the session focused.

Let's say you ask a question about "A," and your client rambles until they end up at "P." If you continue chatting about "P" and the client rambles on from there without any more direction from you, by the end of the session you'll both be so far away from "A" that the conversation won't make any sense. That's the danger of a fully client-led approach.

Instead, you need to co-construct the conversation around the desired outcome. The desired outcome has to be the anchor.

If you think of a therapy conversation as a ship, the ship may have a long chain between "I want to stay sober" and "I want to eat cake," but it's your job to go back to the anchor and ask a connecting question like, "When you eat cake, what do you notice that tells you this isn't a day that you're going to use crystal meth?"

Now the two topics are related. Any follow-up questions should be linked back to the desired outcome as well. The client will have some leeway with the ship's chain, but it's your job to ask, "If we don't wander too far away from the anchor, what do you see, what do you notice, what's different, what's the impact?"

Co-construction is maximizing your clients' autonomy, meaning that they can talk about whatever they want to talk about, but at the same time you're applying your expertise to draw those topics back to the desired outcome.

The entire process is outcome-based, so if you're not talking about what your client really wants to achieve, you're wasting time and the conversation will drift into random irrelevance.

With persistent effort on your part, your client's answers will become focused and less random. They'll realize you're not going to let the desired outcome slide, so they'll eventually stop expressing doubt and hesitation. They'll become more direct and confident. The outcome they describe will no longer feel hypothetical. It will feel real. At that point, the process becomes transformative.

They will be a different person by the time they walk out of therapy.

The "Nevers" List

In doing everything you can to honor and maintain your clients' autonomy and agency, it's useful to remember actions you should *never* take during therapy:

- **Never interpret.** Resist the urge to tell your clients how they should be thinking or feeling about themselves or therapy. The moment you do so, you've disengaged their hearts and minds from the change process. Instead, they're put in a position where they must decide whether they agree with your interpretation, rather than the more empowering act of discovering their own takeaways.

- **Never compliment**. Paying a compliment violates your clients' autonomy because, in receiving a compliment, they are limited to your impression of them, rather than having the choice to discover their own greatness to make changes. Your clients are also likely to reject compliments because it's human nature to avoid being viewed as pompous. The healthy way to pay an "invisible" compliment is to presuppose the best in your clients through the way you ask questions.

- **Never assign homework or tasks**. Doing so steals your clients' authority in their own lives and limits their potential to choose a more powerful course of action. The conversation you co-construct with them during therapy is the intervention they need, not anything you tell them to do.

- **Never strategize**. Your job isn't to problem-solve. Furthermore, dissecting your clients' problems doesn't produce change. Co-constructing their desired outcome produces change. SFBT is all about asking clients to prescribe for themselves what they need in order to become different. They are the experts in their own lives.

- **Never forget your role**. If you really want to help people, you have to learn to get out of their way. Let your clients decide their own process of change. Your job is to apply your expertise through co-construction, which entails structuring therapy sessions around your clients' desired outcome while also using their language—speaking in terms as they describe them—and honoring their agency.

- **Never fix.** Anytime you make a suggestion on how your clients should change, you express some level of doubt in their capability to transform on their own. Inadvertently, you introduce the idea of failure if they don't adhere to what you want them to do.

- **Never summarize the session.** What is meaningful and impactful to you may be different from what is meaningful and impactful to your clients. Summarizing the session dictates how your clients should be digesting therapy, which steals their ownership of the experience.

- **Never let your pride get in the way.** Humility is one of the most underrated skills in SFBT. By being humble, you let the client take center stage. Their progress and their success (or their failure) are their own.

Chapter 6

SFBT Is a Difference-Led Approach

My Most Shocking Session of Therapy

Diving Deep with Elliott

I can't tell you how many times I've been in the middle of a couples' therapy session and have discovered, alongside one of my clients, that something terrible has happened in their relationship.

The most extreme example took place years ago when I was working with a wealthy married couple. Our first session went well, but when I met the husband in the lobby for our second session, he was sitting with his arms crossed, his jaw clenched, and steam jetting out from his ears.

"Is everything okay?" I asked his wife.

She shrugged. "He's been like this for the past few days. I don't know why."

The husband wasn't any more forthcoming, so I proceeded as normal and took the two of them back to my office. "What's been better since we last met?" I asked in the typical way I begin follow-up sessions.

The husband reached into his back pocket, pulled out a folded paper, and opened it. "Before we get into that, look at this." He shoved the paper at me.

A string of expletives raced through my mind as I stared down at what was in my hand: a mug shot of his wife, who had been arrested for prostitution.

She had no idea what was on the piece of paper. Meanwhile, I was suddenly put in the very awkward position of knowing her big secret. *What should I do?* I asked myself. *Hand the paper back to the husband? Give it to the wife?* Once she found out, how would I ever continue therapy?

Out of sheer panic, I placed the piece of paper on my desk and out of sight from the wife. I repeated my question, "So what's been better?"

Clearly, I hadn't followed the script the husband had written for me, so he outed his wife on his own. "That paper is a mug shot from your arrest!" he shouted at her. "I can't believe you didn't tell me what you were doing!"

I'm sure he was thinking, *I've brought you around my wealthy and respected friends, and all the while you've been working as a prostitute!*

The wife burst into tears. Her big secret was now out in the open. As she rattled off some excuses for what she had done, I frantically tried to think of a way to rein in the session. "What's been better?" I asked for the third time.

The husband whirled on me. "Why do you keep asking me that, given what I've just told you?"

I took a steadying breath. "Because you revealed what you did about your wife here, instead of in your living room, so that leads me to think you'd like my help in doing something about it."

"Yeah," he admitted begrudgingly.

"So what's been better?" Four times I'd asked this question now. What allowed me to keep persisting? I believed what I'd just told the husband. I took it as a sign that he wanted his marital relationship to survive because he confronted his wife in my office and not at their home.

He finally answered, "Well, I thought things were going to be pretty okay between us before I discovered this."

"What was going on between you and your wife to let you know things were going pretty okay before you discovered this?" I asked, using his phrasing.

"We were getting along better, connecting better. We were spending more time with one another. We were enjoying ourselves. Don't you agree, honey?" he asked his wife.

My ears perked up. He had just called her *honey*. "So what do we need to do here that helps us overcome your mountain of a problem and get you back to who you were before you discovered this?" I asked.

The husband thought about it. "I'm going to have to find a way to forgive her and have her promise she won't do this anymore."

The wife wiped her wet eyes and added, "And I'm going to have to find a way to earn back his trust and make sure he knows I won't do this anymore."

Now we were getting somewhere. "So let's suppose you forgive at the right rate that works for you," I said to the husband, "and you earn back trust at the right rate that works for you," I said to the wife. "What would you notice?"

The prostitution arrest never came up again for the rest of the session. From that point onward, we were talking about trust, earning trust, forgiveness, and being willing to forgive.

Even though I initially witnessed anger and hurt from this couple—and I myself was shocked because I had never been put in a therapy situation so intense before—I could hear through the husband's pain his desperation for his marriage to succeed. That told me, *Man, you really love this woman.*

With that understanding, I had the confidence to ask difference-making questions that honored what he and his wife really hoped to achieve with their relationship.

The two of them remain married to this day.

The Lens of Difference

Solution focused brief therapy is about difference. Historically, SFBT has been described as a future-focused approach. We don't believe this—SFBT, for us, is a difference-focused approach. In order to do SFBT well, we must remember that we are constantly looking for, asking about, and highlighting (through our questions) signs of difference! In traditional therapy, you're supposed to ask clients questions that help them hash out the root of their problems. But SFBT is a unique approach that requires you to ask questions that highlight what will make a difference in your clients' lives instead.

In the previous example with the married couple, note the questions Elliott asked that kept difference in focus:

- *What's been better since we last met?* In other words, what has been **different** for you?

- *What do we need to do?* In other words, what do we need to do **differently**?

- *What would you notice if you obtained what you wanted?* In other words, what would you identify as **different**?

In SFBT, a therapist's questions are all iterations of difference or change.

Some people criticize SFBT because they say we don't talk about feelings. But if you ask a client about the difference that achieving his best hopes will make and he answers by saying he would feel different, you're going to have an entire conversation about those different feelings.

You might ask, "When you wake up tomorrow as this new version of yourself, what feelings will tell you you're a new person?"

On the other hand, let's say your client isn't a feeling-focused person but a logical processor instead. She might answer your question by saying, "I would think differently." In that case, you're going to have an entire conversation about a different way of thinking.

You might ask, "If this new version of yourself showed up tomorrow, what different thoughts would you be having?"

Another criticism SFBT receives is that it's limited to being only a future-oriented approach, but we also say that's incorrect. It's a difference-oriented approach.

Layers of difference are what you really want to investigate when you say to your client, "Suppose your desired outcome actually shows up. What difference would that make?"

By asking that very simple question, you launch into a conversation that is packed with meaning. If your client gets what she wants, what impact will that have on her? What people in her life would notice the difference? What would be their response? What would those responses mean to her?

While therapy conversations in SFBT all fall under the umbrella of difference and change, they're also guided by the language of your client. You incorporate her language when you ask, "What is different about an experience when you wake up changed?"

In order to incorporate your client's language, you have to learn to listen to them in a new way. In fact, the most important skill you can develop in SFBT is to listen. Changing the way you listen informs the way you talk to your client. Once you start listening differently, you start talking differently, and your client changes. They become different.

In traditional therapy, if a woman says her husband is a jerk, you would need to find out why and how he is a jerk. But in SFBT, you need to listen for the difference in what she's saying instead.

She must really love him, you might think. After all, she's coming to therapy to figure out how to save her relationship, even though she's calling her husband a jerk.

Learn to listen to the hero in the story and let go of your own hero complex (see "Suggestions for Giving Up Power" on page 45). Therapists want to save people, when instead it's more important to make a difference in their lives. You do that by asking questions that highlight the differences your clients would like to experience.

Tips for Listening for the Hero Story

♦ Listen for phrases such as, "It wasn't always like this" or "I used to be so much better," and realize that the strength needed is still inside the client.

♦ Pause to think about why you are impressed with the client, especially since they are dealing with so much.

♦ Think about the client's social location and the ways they have been discriminated against or marginalized. Then think about how they have overcome those experiences in so many ways.

♦ Remember the people in the client's life who love them. Bring all the reasons they might be loved to the forefront of your mind while you formulate each question.

♦ Remember that it takes amazing strength to make it through one day. Each client has done that multiple times before seeing you. Find out how!

By keeping difference in focus, you'll navigate SFBT sessions with clarity and purpose. You'll truly be helpful to your clients.

Difference as Potential Energy

A Closer Look with Adam

In solution focused work, a synonym for *difference* is oftentimes *potential*. As a therapist, your job is to view someone's potential. Asking questions about difference is how you ask what's possible.

"What difference would that make to you?" is our reoccurring question, and in some sense it's another way of asking, *What potential is there for you?*

We don't like using the word *potential* on its own because it means *might or might not*. We don't view our clients as people who might or might not have the ability to change. We view them as fully capable. But *potential* is a good word when it's linked to the idea of energy.

Potential energy is energy that's stored. It already exists. When it converts into something different, it becomes kinetic energy. To go back to synonyms, another word for *potential* is *power*.

There's a power within each person to obtain what they want in life, but that power could go unharnessed. Your job as a therapist is to simply give it a nudge; then that potential energy turns into kinetic energy. Now it's doing what it's supposed to be doing.

Potential energy is like a bow with an arrow nocked and its string pulled back tight. Your client's brilliance—their potential energy—is ready and waiting to be released. They just need to aim and loose the arrow. When that arrow flies, their potential energy changes into kinetic energy. That change-making—that difference—is what solution focused brief therapy is all about.

A change in energy is also connected to the idea of confidence. As a therapist, you need to go into this work with the confidence that you can convert potential energy into kinetic energy. If you attempt therapy with doubts, change isn't going to happen.

Think of therapy as a science experiment in that you need to be the agent of change for a chemical reaction to occur. When it does, kinetic energy will spill out of your client. Transformation will take place.

One More Time for 60 Seconds

Diving Deep with Elliott

In the last year of my undergraduate program, I worked at a treatment center that implemented the 12-step program. One day a new attendee showed up. He kept his hands stuffed in his pockets and lingered in the corner of the room as other people trickled in.

Another guy walked up to him and asked, "Can I help you?" I knew him as someone who was super experienced with these meetings.

"I'm just nervous and scared," the newbie replied. "This is my first time at a twelve-step meeting."

"What are you afraid of?" Mr. Experience asked.

"Losing my kids," the newbie answered frankly. "I've really got to get clean."

I couldn't help but lean in closer. At this time I was 21, and I wasn't sure if I was going to even be a psychotherapist.

"Do me a favor," Mr. Experience told the newbie. "Look at your watch for sixty seconds. Don't do anything else, just stare at it for sixty seconds."

"Okay." The newbie stared at his watch for sixty seconds.

"Can you do that again?" asked Mr. Experience.

"Sure." The newbie did it again.

"One more time for sixty seconds," Mr. Experience said.

The newbie followed through for a third time.

A relaxed smile crossed Mr. Experience's face. "You just proved to yourself that you can stay clean for three minutes. Have a good day." He clapped the newbie on the shoulder and strode away.

I watched what had just happened in amazement. Mr. Experience had treated the newbie as if he were already clean. He recognized his potential energy and gave him the opportunity to demonstrate kinetic energy.

I took away an important lesson from this encounter. The power to change is already within each person. All they have to do is claim it.

The Client's Problem Doesn't Matter

Traditional therapy dictates that you need to dissect your client's problem. They might get worse before they get better, you were taught. We disagree. Why should you attempt to help people change through methods that revolt against the time-honored principles of other professions? Practices of psychotherapy are infantile in comparison.

For example, a good personal trainer will ask you where you want to end up physically. How much do you want to weigh? How much muscle mass do you want to gain? She helps you envision the end result. She doesn't spend a lot of time asking how you got so fat and how long you spent on the couch doing nothing.

The first mistake therapists make when they are learning solution focused brief therapy is that they believe the client's problem matters, when in fact that's irrelevant. The reason a client comes to therapy is that they want something in their life to be different. Once you understand that stance, the obvious first step in the process is to identify what changes the client wants to achieve.

The most generous thing you can do as a therapist is talk to your clients about the outcomes they want as opposed to their diagnoses. You cause harm by stereotyping and stigmatizing when you limit conversations in that way.

Expand the greatness of your clients by viewing them as changeable!

Chapter 7

SFBT Is an Outcome-Led Approach

More Money, More Weed, and More Women

Diving Deep with Elliott

I once conducted a family therapy session with a teenager and his parents. When I asked them what their best hopes were from our talking that day, no one answered. The teenager looked at his parents and shrugged his shoulders.

"Go ahead," they told him. "We're here to be honest."

The teenager met my eyes and lifted his chin. "I want more money, more weed, and more women," he said. Instead of *women*, however, he used an expletive I'm not going to repeat.

Obviously his reply wasn't a desired outcome the parents could buy into, and family therapy requires establishing an outcome that works for everyone present, so I asked, "What else would you like?"

"I want my parents to get off my back," he snapped.

That still wasn't an agreeable outcome for everyone, so I asked again, "What else would you like to achieve from coming here?"

Unexpectedly, the teenager's lips started to quiver. "I want my parents to believe in me," he confessed, his eyes welling with tears.

Not only did his answer shock me, given how poorly he had been behaving, but it also was an outcome that the whole family could agree on. It allowed me to ask, "Suppose you woke up tomorrow and you were behaving in a way that gave your parents an easier time believing in you, what would you notice?"

In a touching way, the teenager started to describe what he wanted his parents to see in him. He conveyed that, even though he hadn't made great decisions in his life, he was trying to do better.

Through our continued conversation, he revealed that he had always wanted to work with his dad, who made a good living. He hoped he could take over his dad's company one day. A large part of why he had been acting out stemmed from his father not giving him the opportunity to learn the business.

What on the surface had looked like defiance was in reality just teenage frustration.

As the parents also shared their thoughts, our conversation deepened to include what they needed their son to do to help them believe he was headed in the right direction.

I met with this family three times in total. The second time was to check on their progress, which was notable. During our third session, when I asked how things were going, the teenager replied, "Your job sucks!"

Oh, no, I thought. He was being disrespectful again. I thought we'd moved past that roadblock.

"When I drove here with my parents before our first session," the teenager continued, "they told me I'd be seeing you for years, as long as was necessary. But this is our last appointment. If you had just kept on seeing me, my dad would have paid you forever. He's loaded! But because of the way you do therapy, you're never going to see me again."

I couldn't help laughing. "Yep, you're right, man. My job sucks." My response was tongue-in-cheek, however, because I have the best job in the world. This teenager and his parents were proof. They had been changed in only three visits.

Besides, this teenager didn't know something I did: my office was flooding with referrals from his dad, who had been telling his friends, "My kid is on his way to a bright and positive future, and this psychotherapist Elliott helped it happen!"

One of the coolest things about solution focused brief therapy is that people share their success with others, which helps your practice thrive. In this case, the dad was able to tell people, "After only three sessions, I got my son back."

What a gift it was to be a part of that.

The Power of Hope

In addition to solution focused brief therapy being a difference-led approach, it's also an outcome-led approach. When we speak of outcomes, what we really mean is "the desired outcome the client wants to achieve."

Desired outcome isn't the language we recommend using with clients, however. It's better to speak in more conversational terms by asking them about their "best hopes."

Your clients' desired outcome is the target you're aiming for in each therapy session, and because *desired outcome* is synonymous with *best hope*, SFBT can also be thought of as a hope-led approach. Your clients' best hopes are always the focus of your session.

Transformation is another word we've also started interchanging with *desired outcome*, because when you ask your clients to reveal their best hopes, you're essentially asking, "What changes are you hoping to achieve?" In other words, "What will be different—what transformation will occur—if you live consistently with your best hope?"

Transformation happens when hope takes root and continues to flourish. Hope is that driver of change. It must be at the foundation of every question you ask. Those questions need to have built into them the presupposition of belief in your clients, even in the face of significant challenges.

When you ask, "What is your best hope?" and your client answers, "I don't know," don't give up! Instead you might ask, "Can you take a little time right now to think about it so that you might know?" or "Can you tell me what you *do* know?"

At other times, your clients might say their best hope is something grand and amazing. In that case, don't diminish their hopes by replying, "Can you think of something more realistic?"

Communicate faith in their competency. Believe in them every step of the way.

Remember that when you believe your clients are capable of anything, they start acting as if they're capable of anything. They transform.

Hope and the Human Brain

A Closer Look with Adam

Hope is healing, and that healing effect on the brain is measurable and tangible. Trauma, on the other hand, is destructive.

When people experience trauma, their hippocampus is impacted and has a difficult time distinguishing between past, present, and future. Consequently, when they experience a flashback, they can't determine whether their trauma is currently happening or if it happened in the past. To make matters worse, their amygdala starts flooding with fear, worry, and stress.

Hope is the remedy.

"What is your best hope?" is an essential question because it leads to a hope-filled conversation. Hope-filled conversations are dynamic; they allow the brain to get better at distinguishing past, present, and future. Distinguishing the future, in turn, enables your clients to open their minds to new possibilities, simply because the amygdala is now flooding the hippocampus with hope, optimism, and joy.

Your clients will change right before you. The answers they may have given at the beginning of the session will become different as well. SFBT is that transformative. It's evidence-based and remarkable and laser-focused on hope.

Think of the example Elliott shared with the teenager who initially said his best hopes were to get more weed, more money, and more women. When Elliott asked what else he wanted, the teenager replied, "I want my parents to get off my back."

Those first two answers might have conveyed defiance, but Elliott persisted by asking again, "What else do you want?"

Do you see how his question was filled with hope? It was synonymous with asking, "What else are you hoping for?"

The teenager's final answer was something Elliott, and perhaps the boy's mom and dad, never saw coming: "I want my parents to believe in me." That was his true best hope, and it took Elliott asking the same question three times—with hope—in order to get him to answer from the heart.

Once the teenager's meaningful outcome was established, Elliott was able to spend the rest of the session co-constructing a description of that best hope. He asked questions like, "How would your parents show you they believe in you?" and "What difference would it make to know they believe in you?" and "How would you let them know you were so pleased to see them believe in you?"

Belief is powerful. When people believe in themselves, they become capable of anything. Your job is to honor that belief, even when your client struggles to see hope in the moment.

Now imagine you were the therapist working with this teenager. You could sympathize with his challenge—lean into the emotion of it—by asking, "Even on your hardest days, when it might be difficult for your parents to believe in you, what would let you know their belief was still present?"

Do you see how hope can be derived by making a contrast from the worst, the most painful, and the most difficult challenge to the most hopeful outcome?

Be diligent about creating language that is hope-filled. Insert your client's desired outcome into the contrast of their challenge. That's how hope grows and becomes an agent of change. Once you master hopeful language, you'll listen in amazement as your client articulates powerful and hopeful answers.

Earn Your Client's Answers

Solution focused brief therapy isn't client-led; it's outcome-led. In order to help your clients achieve their desired outcomes, you have to keep pushing when you hit a roadblock. If your clients don't know what their best hopes are, or if they begin by answering flippantly, keep persisting, because SFBT happens on the other side of those meaningful best hopes. Without them, the session breaks apart.

Special Note about the Word *Meaningful*

You may have noticed already, but the word *meaningful* is an adjective we use regularly when describing the details of the clients' desired outcome and accompanying description. We aren't just trying to get any old details or any old desired outcome. Rather, we are trying to understand what motivates clients, what clients are passionate about, what their "why" is for everything they do. When we access these meaningful details, the descriptions become change-motivating. SFBT therapists must work to get meaningful details.

You know you have meaningful details when one or more of the following occurs:

♦ The client gets excited about the answer(s) they are giving.

♦ Their face lights up and they think about something they haven't realized before.

♦ They mention people who touch their heart in a special way (like partners, parents, children, or close friends).

♦ They cry happy tears about the details they're sharing.

♦ They link the details to the best version of themselves.

With enough persistence and belief from you, your clients will declare their best hopes, but oftentimes their honest answers will only come after a show of defense mechanisms. After all, life has taught them that stating what they hope for will be met with disbelief, criticism, and mockery.

People have warned them that what they want will be hard to achieve, so they should prepare for disappointment or even quit while they still can, and that answer has crushed them.

As a therapist, you have to earn the right to hear your clients' answers. They have to believe that sharing their hopes will be met with faith and not doubt.

When they say, "I don't know what my best hopes are," what they really mean is, "I'm not sure I'm brave enough to tell you." Your job is to earn their answer. Don't let yourself believe your clients are resistant, difficult, or incapable. They're just scared and they don't know you, while the people they do know have stomped on their goals.

Give them a minute if they can't answer right away. Let them develop the ability to be brave.

Once they state what their best hopes are, that hope will become transformative. Declaring a goal can be scary, however, and you have to let people build up the courage to get there in your office.

Don't give up on pushing for a meaningful best hope. If you do, you make it that much easier for your clients to give up on themselves. They'll default to living their lives based on their limitations and not their potential.

Show your clients you are trustworthy by allowing them enough space and time to learn that you'll wait for their genius to shine in their answers.

Chapter 8

Presuppose the Best in Your Client

The "Bad" Student

Diving Deep with Elliott

My previous battles with depression helped me develop the skill to presuppose the best in others. Growing up, I wished influential people had viewed me in the best light possible when in reality they viewed me in the worst.

During my high school years, I rarely did my homework. Consequently, my teachers and administrators determined I wasn't a good student or studious by nature. They labeled me as unintelligent, even though I scored high every time I took their intelligence tests. Despite that, I was still treated like a bad student and kept getting kicked out of class.

When I walked into my math classroom, my teacher would ask, "Elliott, do you have your homework?" I would answer, "No." He would say, "Go sit in the office."

I spent the majority of my freshman year doing math homework in the vice principal's office. I'm sure it wouldn't surprise you to learn that math never became my strong suit.

Instead of judging me, I wished someone would have asked, "Why don't you do your math homework?" I would have answered, "Because my dad beats me up."

When he found out I hadn't done my math homework yet, he beat me, so I learned to tell lies. "I've already done my math homework," I'd say, only to have him beat me up for rushing through it. I learned to tell a different lie: "I'm going to do it later so I can focus." That didn't work either; he'd beat me for not taking it seriously. The only trick that worked was to not mention my math homework at all. And if I didn't do it, I just didn't do it.

I used to set my alarm clock for two in the morning because it was the safest time to do my homework. Everyone in the house was asleep by then. Sometimes I was able to wake up and work for one or two hours. Sometimes I accidentally slept through my alarm clock and didn't get any work done.

As an adult looking back now, I'm able to see that the person I've just described—a boy who was willing to wake up at 2 A.M. to do his homework—seems like a very studious person. Unfortunately, everyone treated me like I didn't respect homework or that I didn't take academics seriously.

I came to believe I was stupid, because when enough people tell you you're dumb, you eventually believe it.

What helped me become the way I am now was wishing someone had looked at me with more perspective—like there was a justifiable reason for what was going on, like I actually had a strength instead of just a problem.

After all, I had found a way to protect myself from my father's beatings. True, it came at the cost of my high school academics, but I did find a way to keep myself safe.

How did I change from being a "C student" in high school to an "A student" in college? I met a professor, Dr. Michael Ellison, who caused me to doubt my perceived truth about myself.

"You're a very good writer," he told me one day. "Where did you learn how to write like that?"

I stared at him blankly, taken aback. "I didn't know I was a good writer."

He took me into his office and said, "Elliott, I have to be honest with you. The one part of my job I hate is grading papers. I feel like I'm reading the same papers over and over again. But there's something different about your papers. When I get to the end of them, I find myself wishing there was more. As someone who doesn't like grading, that's very rare for me."

I couldn't believe what I was hearing. Slowly, the fog of negativity in which I had viewed myself started to clear. When we finished speaking, I didn't walk out of my professor's office convinced of my own brilliance as a writer, but I did walk away doubting the reality that I was dumb.

As an SFBT practitioner, you need to give your clients that same constructive form of doubt. In other words, you need to demonstrate faith in them. The only way to do that is by arguing their reality. Your primary job is to help people see themselves in a new and kinder light.

Learn to think past a client's problem by asking yourself, "What strength is hiding within this person?" When you do that—when you see your clients through a prism of strength—you give them a tremendous gift.

For the record, I graduated college with a 4.0 GPA and later did the same while working toward my Ph.D. I trace the pivot point of my success back to my early college professor who saw the best in me.

Find the Hero in the Story

Have you ever heard the language *Solution Focused Brief Therapy 1.0* versus *2.0*? A good friend of ours, Mark McKergow, a scientist and international consultant, wrote an article (McKergow, 2016) in which he identified multiple versions of SFBT that he highlighted as 1.0 versus 2.0. What was the biggest difference between them? The use of presuppositions.

We would take that one step further and argue that the biggest difference is actually how language is used, and presuppositions are one way to achieve that.

A presupposition is a linguistic tool that makes an assumption that is related to the conversation in which the truth of the assumption is taken for granted by the speaker.

If you want to evoke change in a client, you should put that change into language. And the easiest way for you to do that is through presuppositions.

If a client tells you she wants to become a French chef, it behooves you to presuppose that she can do it, as opposed to asking, "Can you do it?" The latter leaves the window open for her to answer, "No."

Now imagine the same client says, "I want to be a French chef, but I'm allergic to butter." A lot of therapists would respond by saying, "You're going to have a hard time being a French chef because French cooking requires a lot of butter."

The better course of action is to presuppose that your client has found a way to overcome her obstacle.

Elliott might say instead, "Suppose you are traveling home from France after officially being made a French chef. How pleased would you be to know that you have found a way to cook around your butter allergy?"

Maintaining the belief that any client can overcome her obstacle and achieve the outcome she desires is presupposing in action.

"Find the hero in the story" is our mantra. And as an SFBT therapist, you need to learn to do the same. You'll become better at this work when you allow yourself to be amazed by people. Practice this skill in your everyday life, even in simple moments such as watching TV, reading a book, or interacting with others on social media.

When Elliott was watching *Chopped*, an American TV cooking competition show, one of the competitors stood out to him. She was a vegan chef, and during one episode she was given meat that she was required to use in a recipe.

Staying true to her vegan lifestyle, she didn't taste the meat as she prepared it, but as a result she didn't know if her dish was seasoned well. She found a work-around.

After cooking the meat, she cut off a small piece and ran it over to one of the other chefs to ask if he would taste-test it for her. He did and told her it needed a little more salt. She added more and asked him to taste it again. This time he said it was perfect.

Elliott saw two heroes in that episode: the vegan who found a way to solve her problem, and the contestant who helped her, even though he didn't gain any advantage by doing so.

Go through your life like this, looking for the heroes in people. Look for strengths in your clients when it's easier to see their problems. Practice believing there is no such thing as a flaw—there is nothing wrong with anyone you've ever met in your life.

Listen Through, Talk Through, and Believe In

As human beings, we're trained to believe that what other people tell us is correlated to the truth, even when it's demeaning. SFBT practitioners often struggle to build the skill of presupposing the best in their clients because it violates that instinct as a human.

Presupposing the best in someone is an important skill to develop, however, because what you hear from your client and the truth are often incongruent.

How many times have you heard a client describe himself with a negative label or a derogatory blanket statement?

"I'm a terrible father."

"I'm incapable of making friends."

"I can't stay sober."

It happens all the time, and yet these statements are rarely true. At the very least, they don't convey the full truth.

Elliott once had a client who started to weep and said, "I'm such a failure. All I do is fail."

That's strange, Elliott thought to himself. *If all you've ever done in your life is fail, I don't know how you got to be in your forties.*

"What do you do for a living?" Elliott asked him.

"I'm a lawyer," he replied.

Hmm, Elliott thought. *That doesn't fit with your self-diagnosis of "I've only ever failed."* It was incongruent with the truth.

"How did you become a lawyer?" Elliott asked.

"Oh, that was easy."

Was it? "How did you find it easy?"

"My grandfather is a judge," the man went on. "My grand-mother is a lawyer. My mother is also a judge, and my dad is also a lawyer. It's just what we do in my family."

He wasn't taking any credit for his success.

"Slow down for a second," Elliott said. "You are now describing something as easy that a lot of people experience as hard. As a matter of fact, the average dropout rate of law school is greater than fifty percent. So how did you become one of the other fifty percent who made it through?"

The conversation shifted, and the man began to see himself in a new light. He started taking credit for the skills that made him special.

When we talk about presupposition, we often use phrases such as "listening through," "talking through," and "believing in."

We "listen through" a client's untrue words to what they're really trying to express. We "talk through" a client's negative image of themselves to the best version of themselves. We "believe in" a client rather than believing their statements of self-doubt. We believe in the hero in them, the person who can achieve what they desire most in life.

To put it plainly, we seek out someone's heart, and we speak to it.

When we ask questions that presuppose people are awe-some, they answer from a place of awesomeness, greatness, and confidence.

For example, Elliott often asks the couples he works with, "Tell me about the best date you've ever been on together."

Did you catch the presuppositions within that statement? He presupposed the couple has been on a date together, that they have enjoyed at least one of those dates, and that they can recall that specific date right now.

He didn't ask, "Have you ever gone on a date together that you enjoyed?" He said, "Tell me about the best one."

A presupposition means assuming positive information, even though you shouldn't already know it. Presuppositions also tend to include "invisible compliments."

You're paying a compliment when you say, "Tell me about the best date you've been on together." You're assuming that since your clients are in a relationship, they wouldn't have entered into it without experiencing some spark of attraction and compatibility. That's praiseworthy.

Presuppositions manifest the extraordinarily strong communication of belief. And belief allows the client to articulate how transformation can be a reality.

Argue without Offending

As we mentioned earlier, presupposing the best in people runs counter to how we've been conditioned as humans. We're inclined to accept the answers they give us at face value. We're also prone to believe we shouldn't accuse them of telling falsehoods.

Imagine you asked a woman where she bought her glasses and she answered, "The thrift store." If you went on to call her a liar, she would likely be offended. But SFBT requires you to argue with your clients' version of the truth. The trick is to do so in a way that doesn't cause offense.

Let's say a man tells you, "I'm not that wonderful." You need to reply by saying something like, "Huh, so you're not that wonderful. Who in your life would argue with that?"

If he answers, "My wife," you might say, "If I ask your wife why she thinks you're so wonderful, what do you think she would tell me?"

Good therapy changes a client's truth, so you have to be willing to argue about that truth.

In the scenario above, you should want the man to walk out of therapy at least doubting his perceived truth of "I'm not that wonderful." Ideally, you also want him thinking, *Maybe I am that wonderful.*

Presuppositions Can Offer Sympathy and Encouragement

Solution focused brief therapy is often criticized as a Band-Aid approach, meaning it just skims the surface of addressing a client's pain or hardship. We disagree.

Through presuppositions, we have endless opportunities to offer sympathy and encouragement, while at the same time keeping our therapy sessions focused on a client's desired outcome and the difference it would make in their life, rather than dissecting their problem, which doesn't produce change.

The magic of presuppositions is that it can highlight how challenging a hardship is while also instilling confidence in a client.

As a therapist, you might ask, "Given that you're facing this difficulty on a regular basis, how are you the kind of person who continues to push forward?"

That question has the underlying message, *I understand that this obstacle is hard for you, but I have complete faith in your ability to overcome it.*

By asking a question with a positive presupposition embedded, we co-construct a competent, confident, capable version of the client. This is the transformed version of the client that they came to therapy to find.

Mentally Healthy People Own Their Strengths

Another way we are trained as human beings is to restrain from bragging about ourselves. People often say to Elliott, "When you were a kid, you were really great at baseball."

His instinct is to reply, "Yeah, it was just my thing."

But the truth is that a lot of people can't hit a baseball. That's a skill. It's something Elliott should own, just like he does with his other talents.

We want people to take credit for their own skills, and we challenge ourselves to make sure they do so. In therapy, presupposing the best in your client is your avenue to get that conversation started.

Elliott's favorite rapper is Jay-Z, and back in 2008, Jay-Z was the first hip-hop artist to headline the Glastonbury Festival in the U.K. A lot of people criticized the festival's organizers for featuring a rapper, and the loudest critic was former headliner Noel Gallagher, lead guitarist and co-lead singer of the band Oasis.

"I'm sorry, but Jay-Z? No chance," Noel complained. "Glastonbury has the tradition of guitar music . . . I'm not having hip-hop at Glastonbury. It's wrong."

Jay-Z addressed Noel's protests in an interview with the magazine *Bizarre*. "We have to respect each other's genre of music and move forward," he said. "I've never ever had a show that's caused this much of a stir, so I'm really looking forward to it."

What Jay-Z went on to do at the Glastonbury Festival speaks volumes. He walked out on stage with a guitar strapped around him—an instrument he barely plays—and he opened his set with a performance of Oasis's hit song, "Wonderwall."

Some of the audience sang along. Most of them chanted Jay-Z's name.

"For those that didn't get the memo," the rapper shouted, "my name is Jay-Z, and I'm pretty f***ing awesome."

What makes people like Jay-Z so amazing is that they claim their strengths. As human beings, we are trained to claim our flaws instead, and then we're rewarded by people who tell us we're humble. But in order to be mentally healthy, you have to claim your zones of genius—and it isn't arrogant to do so.

If Elliott's friend asked him to fix his car and Elliott answered, "Sure, I can figure that out," that would be arrogant because Elliott can't even change a tire. Instead, Elliott should say, "I don't think I'm the person you should be asking, but I can give you the names of people who might be able to help."

On the other hand, if Elliott's friend were to ask, "Are you any good at solution focused brief therapy?" Elliott has every justification to answer, "Yeah, I'm pretty f***ing awesome." After all, SFBT is in the wheelhouse of things he does well. It's his zone of genius.

Confident people own their strengths. Likewise, mentally healthy people own their weaknesses. Elliott is fine to tell people, "I'm a very bad wrench turner, but I'm a really good check writer." He'll gladly pay someone to fix his car, and he can do so without shame.

As an SFBT practitioner, you need to help people discover their own zones of genius. Every person you've ever met has one, even if they're using that zone of genius for bad.

People get enough grief from the world pointing out how horrible they are. What they need—and what the world rarely offers—is pointing out how amazing they are.

You have the great privilege to be a positive voice for your clients, and you can do that by asking questions that help them identify their own brilliance.

Train your brain to think in a new way. Live your life believing that what people are good at is awesome, and what they're not good at is irrelevant.

Chapter 9

Trust Your Client's Capability

The Fighting Couple Versus the Sparkling Couple

Diving Deep with Elliott

No one's life is perfect. If you accept that as true, then you must also accept that no one's life is perfectly imperfect. Every person with a great life has some flaw or challenge, which also means every person with a flawed or challenging life has some perfection.

As a solution focused therapist, you can't allow yourself to think, "Can I really help clients who have never experienced peace or romance or love? What about couples who have never smiled together?"

I've worked with couples who have claimed they've never been close. *Really?* I thought. *You have three children in my office right now who are making a bunch of noise.* That couple must have gotten close at least three times.

People talk in absolutes when they don't actually mean *absolutely.* They're just trying to convey the difficulty of their circumstances.

A few years ago, I worked with a lesbian couple, Jen and Deja (names changed), who had a very volatile relationship. We had a wonderful first session of therapy together, but when they came back for their second session, they seemed as if they had taken a step back.

I asked what had been better since the last time we met, and they looked absolutely deflated.

"We left our last appointment with you on cloud nine," Jen said, "but then two days later we started fighting again. We've been fighting ever since. That sparkling moment was over."

As I believed in them rather than believing how they were defining themselves as the fighting couple, I said, "In the week before you came to your first session of therapy, how many days did you fight?"

"Seven," Deja answered. "The entire week."

"So after one session of therapy, how many days did you experience fighting in the following week?"

"Five," Deja replied.

"What role did you two play after walking out of that session that reduced the days you spent fighting from seven to five?"

Deja looked at Jen thoughtfully. "Well, we talked about how amazing therapy was and how good it felt to hear hopeful things come out of each other's mouths. But then two days later we slipped up."

"All right," I said. "Suppose that when you left my office today, you went from five days fighting to four-and-a-half days fighting. What would you notice?"

The tone of our conversation shifted. They began to see what they'd failed to recognize before.

"Wow," Jen said. "We were so focused on the five wrong days we spent as a fighting couple that we didn't notice the two good days we were a sparkling couple."

"A lot of couples wouldn't be able to create two good days," Deja added, "and we did."

In that moment, they redefined their relationship. All of a sudden, they weren't the fighting couple; they weren't the couple that failed. They were the couple who had succeeded in creating two good days.

People say things like, "I don't know how to be in a healthy relationship." In response, you have to think, *Yeah, you do. You've just been hurt, and it's your hurt that's talking now.*

People also ask me, "Elliott, how do you believe someone can succeed in achieving their desired outcome?" My answer is, "Because they wouldn't be in my office if they didn't know how to do it."

It's my job to help my clients illuminate the answer that's already inside them. And the best way to do that is by listening through the problem, not to the problem.

If you can learn how to do that, you can learn how to master SFBT with anyone. As a matter of fact, developing that skill will make you a better parent, a better spouse, a better employee, and an all-around better person.

When I hear from a client, "I feel like the world is crashing in on me," I can't help but think of how that reflects the best in her. As I listen through, I recognize she must be really strong to deal with that feeling of the world crashing in on her.

If you want to help people, you have to inspire them to redefine themselves. The way they see themselves in their own eyes is directly related to their ability to change.

Become Allergic to Doubt and Fear

Trusting your clients' capability goes hand in hand with presupposing the best in them. Trusting your clients' capability is part of that stance we talked about at the beginning of the book, and this stance of belief manifests in the language we use. Presuppositions are one behavioral manifestation where we are holding that stance. Our clients should feel our belief in them because that belief is built into the presuppositional questions we ask. As a solution focused therapist, you need to talk to your clients as if they're capable of change—capable of living life differently. It's a given that all clients want change, so you need to talk about change, and you need to talk to your clients as if they can achieve change.

Think about parents who are teaching their child how to tie a shoe. Inevitably, the child will get frustrated and say, "I can't do this!" The child will try to persuade them their child is not a shoe tier.

The parents still have faith that, although their child isn't a shoe tier yet, the child has the capability to become a shoe tier. They say things that convey a belief that the child can be different:

"You can do it."

"Let me show you one more time, and then you try again."

"What is the first step?"

"Now where do you put your fingers next?"

They talk him through a change process. They don't believe him when he says, "I can't do it."

Your clients behave in a similar way as this child. When they come into your office, they try to persuade you that for whatever reason they're not capable of change.

It's your job to believe *in* them and not believe their statements of doubt. See a better version of them. Maybe they're not changed yet, but they have the capability to change.

Faith is required in order to do this work. When therapists listen to their clients' doubts and fears, the tendency is to also behave from a position of doubt and fear. Instead, refuse to attend to corrosive thoughts and attitudes. It will set you apart as a therapist.

Elliott likes to say he's allergic to doubt and fear.

Develop that same allergy. It's the best kind to have.

Believe in the Journey

Diving Deep with Elliott

Adam has three children, and I am good friends with Adam's son, Toby, whom I like to call my homie.

Toby is a brilliant kid who often gets bored with school because it comes so easily to him. Sometimes Adam worries that if Toby doesn't perform at his best, he won't get into a great college. But if Adam were to start behaving from a position of doubt and fear, that would be detrimental to Toby.

Now let's say Adam came to me for therapy. My job would be to restore Adam's language to faith and not fear. I would ask things like, "What are you hoping for Toby to achieve?" and "What difference would it make for Toby to achieve these things?"

By the end of the conversation, Adam should be saying things like, "You know what? So what if Toby doesn't go to my top pick for a college? He might go to some other good school instead. And you know what? Maybe Toby would rather go to a trade school to become a mechanic."

He starts believing in Toby's journey.

We get hundreds of e-mails a month from therapists asking if solution focused brief therapy can help clients who are dealing with trauma, personality disorders, drug addictions, you name it. We have the same response to each of them: "Do you hear the doubt you're expressing?"

Sensitize yourself to doubt. Believe in your client's capability to change. Believe in your own capability to evoke change.

SFBT can help anyone. Trust in yourself and your client and the process.

The Tip to Flip

A Closer Look with Adam

Let's say you have a client who insists on telling you the details of their problem, and you don't know how to steer the conversation back on course. Listen through the problem for something positive about the client, and use it to pivot the conversation.

Perhaps in elaborating on the client's problem, your client says they're nervous about their kids. Inwardly recognize that her nervousness means the client cares about their kids and wants the best for them.

Instead of asking what makes the client so nervous, flip that question by presupposing the opposite of nervous. In other words, presuppose the best in your client.

You might ask, "If you could keep your kids safe (if you could presuppose the flipped state of your problem), what difference would you notice in yourself?"

There's no need to waste time asking a bunch of questions about the reverse state of the problem in an effort to transition the conversation back on track. You can just flip the conversation by presupposing that it's flipped. Once you do that, you begin talking to the version of the client who is capable of flipping it.

As you listen to your clients' problems, presuppose the best traits in them. Those might be confidence, competence, capability, and strength. Learn to listen so well that you find those pivot points faster.

Focus your time on speaking to the best version of your client.

Don't Set a Bar

Randy Pausch, a computer science professor at Carnegie Mellon University, was told he had three to six months to live following a recurrence of pancreatic cancer. In 2007, one month after receiving his diagnosis, he gave a lecture at CMU called "Really Achieving Your Childhood Dreams," which became the Internet sensation known as "The Last Lecture."

When a professor at Carnegie Mellon University retires, he or she gives a last lecture, an event in a large auditorium that is recorded live. Randy was an especially beloved professor who had to retire early because of his terminal illness, and his last lecture was packed with attendees.

One of the things Randy talked about was the course he'd developed for undergraduates in which he taught them how to build virtual worlds.

There had never been a course like it before. It entailed 50 students working in randomly chosen teams of four. Those teams were given two weeks to build a virtual reality experience. After sharing their projects, the students were then shuffled into new groups of four before starting again, building new virtual reality experiences. This process was repeated for the duration of the semester.

When the time came for the students to share their first two-week projects, the virtual reality worlds that they created blew Randy away. Their work was spectacular and went far beyond what he thought undergraduates could achieve.

It left him at a loss for how to continue to guide them. He had been a professor for 10 years at this point, and never before had he seen this level of work from his students.

Seeking advice, Randy called his mentor, Andy van Dam, who had been his professor at Brown University.

"Andy, I just gave [my students] a two-week assignment," Randy said, "and they came back and did stuff that, if I'd given them a whole semester [to complete], I would have given them all A's. What should I do?"

Andy thought for minute and answered, "You go back to class tomorrow, and you look them in the eye and say, 'Guys, that was pretty good, but I know you can do better.'"

That was wonderful advice because Randy didn't know where to set the bar with his students, and he was only going to do them a disservice by setting it at all.

The act of setting a bar, whether high or low, was a limitation.

Randy followed his mentor's advice, and his students went on to excel even more. Their peers, friends, and even parents came to see them showcase their virtual worlds. Soon they had to use a big auditorium to fit all the attendees, and even then people stood in the back and in the aisles just to squeeze in and watch.

Randy went on to teach this groundbreaking course for the next 10 years, and he never set a bar for his students.

As a solution focused therapist, Elliott has worked countless times with clients who are struggling with serious addictions or debilitating mental illnesses, and he doesn't know where to set the bar with them. Instead, like Randy, he's developed a discipline to not set a bar.

Sometimes his clients come back and say they haven't touched alcohol for a week. If Elliott had set a bar for them, he might have just asked them to stay sober for a day. But because he didn't, they did something that exceeded his expectations.

An intervention in therapy is a limitation because it inherently sets a bar, and we have developed a discipline to let our clients set the bar instead. If it's low, great. We'll deal with that as we continue therapy. If it's high, great. We'll deal with that as we continue therapy.

Setting a bar is a limiting act when you don't know a person's capability. And when do you ever really know someone's capability? Instead, we have chosen to not take limiting acts in our approach to SFBT. The outcome of psychotherapy should be limitless.

Achievable Outcomes

"Talk therapy" is much more effective than we give it credit for, and solution focused brief therapy is a very effective form of talk therapy.

Practitioners have a tendency to think, *Oh, my client is dealing with a real problem right now, so talk therapy won't work.* But that's not true. The research doesn't support that. The American Psychological Association clarifies that psychotherapy is not only effective but also oftentimes produces larger effects than many other medical treatments, including medication (American Psychological Association, 2012). Talk therapy helps with real problems.

Keep in mind that psychotherapy isn't always about fixing the stated problem, though. We're aware we can't fix a terminal illness, for example. What we can do is have an impact on the way our clients live their lives when facing significant difficulties.

Elliott worked with several clients who had moved to Fort Worth, Texas, from New Orleans to escape the flooding from Hurricane Katrina. This was during his internship program for graduate school, and many of his colleagues doubted SFBT could help these people, especially when their desired outcome was wishing Hurricane Katrina had never happened.

Elliott will never forget one of his clients, Grace (name changed). When Elliott asked Grace what her best hopes were from their talking together, she told him a horrific story about how when she was in the flood, the raging water ripped her grandchild from her arms. She wasn't sure if she would ever see that grandchild again.

Even though Grace didn't answer Elliott's best-hopes question directly, it was clear to him that she wanted her grandchild back—something beyond his ability to help her achieve. So instead he asked her, "How do you know you're strong enough to get through this challenge? How do you know you can handle whatever is coming next?"

Grace answered, "Because I've been through difficult times in my past."

"What things did you draw upon to get through those difficult times?" Elliott asked.

They went on to have a conversation about her capability to endure difficult times.

Your job is to ask questions about attainable outcomes, especially as they relate to the restraints of your occupation. If you were a medical doctor and a client asked you to cure her terminal illness, you might have a different answer. But as a solution focused therapist, your role is to talk about desired outcomes—transformations—and how to achieve those outcomes.

PART III

The Diamond

Chapter 10

Introducing the Diamond Model

The diamond model is one of the biggest innovations in the field of solution focused brief therapy. It's a flowchart that comprises the five skills you need to master to do solution focused brief therapy effectively. It guides you through every moment of a session, so you'll never get lost in a session again. You'll know with absolute clarity where you are, where you've been, and what comes next.

The Need for the Diamond

Therapists go to school for years to study psychotherapy, but they soon discover that learning theory is very different from putting it into practice. As a result, they worry about not knowing what to do in sessions with their clients.

Adam tells therapists, "I should be able to pause you at any moment in a session and say, 'Why did you ask that question?'" Ninety percent of the time, they have no idea. Their answers are vague iterations of "It was just a question that felt good in the moment."

That isn't going to cut it in an era where insurance companies and third-party payers are only willing to pay for evidence-based approaches that are backed by research. Most importantly, if you don't know what you're doing, you can't do it well. Research shows that when clients see competent therapists, they get better.

Helping people is why you got into this field, but you're not being helpful if you get lost in a session, if you can't defend your approach, and if you don't know how to guide your clients through a meaningful change process.

We created the diamond model in an effort to help therapists understand how to be as helpful and as effective as possible within their clinical work. We want to help as many clients as possible, and we can do that through you—by teaching you how to master this approach through the diamond.

Evolving from the Art Gallery Metaphor

We had been working together for several years before we started developing the diamond. Until then, we believed Chris Iveson had come up with the best explanation of what should happen during a therapy session. Chris made an analogy to an art gallery. Before you go into an art gallery, you have to obtain a ticket. Establishing your clients' best hopes (their desired outcome) is your ticket.

Once you have that ticket, you go into the resource talk room, where you get to know your clients. The purpose there is to learn your clients' language so you know how to speak to them.

From that point, you go into the main attraction of the art gallery, the preferred future (something we now call "future of the outcome," which we will talk more about later), where you spend most of your time. In order to have a meaningful experience in the preferred future, however, you get to know your clients a little better so you can ask them meaningful questions about their desired outcome.

Finally, in order to leave the art gallery, you need to go through the gift shop—in other words, the closing of your session. But because what is in that gift shop is only a cheap imitation of what you've already seen and spent your time doing, your aim should be exiting the gift shop as quickly as possible so that you do not ruin the experience you've had in the main attraction.

Chris Iveson's perspective of closing was a departure from how Steve de Shazer and Insoo Kim Berg had been practicing SFBT decades earlier. They put a lot of focus on the end of a session. Before the session ended, they would take a break and discuss the session with their team of therapists. The team would then create a task for the client, which the main therapist would relay upon returning.

Our view of closing falls mostly in line with the gift shop metaphor. We believe it's not our job to assign a task, summarize the session, or pay compliments to our clients, because those are only cheap imitations of what they should be taking away on their own.

In the first several years that we practiced SFBT, we conducted our sessions and taught using the art gallery approach, but as we continued to analyze other solution focused professionals, we became more conflicted about whether the art gallery was an all-inclusive explanation of therapy.

Current practitioners in our field, such as the brilliant team of therapists at BRIEF in the U.K., implemented SFBT in various ways. Harvey Ratner hated the preferred future (detailing with the client what they would like for their future) and spent a lot of time doing scales (numerically identifying the details of change). Chris Iveson predominantly fixated on the preferred future, while Evan George tended to focus on resource talk (details within the client that could be utilized to produce change).

Although we learned a lot from studying other professionals, we became increasingly frustrated that the masters of this approach were all practicing what they called SFBT but then executing it in substantially different ways. In an effort to help practitioners become good at SFBT, we took it upon ourselves to simplify and clarify the solution focused approach. By helping other therapists, we could help more clients get better service. And helping people is our number one priority. And it's what led us to create the diamond.

The Three-Step Process of the Diamond

Before we created the diamond, we put in countless hours of research and study about SFBT. We spent countless hours reviewing recorded therapy. We analyzed how the most experienced long-term professionals were practicing this approach. We literally traveled the world to interview these people. We even conducted a Delphi study before we came up with the diamond. This is not a random idea. This came after a decade of careful work.

At first, we looked for what each clinician was doing differently, but at a certain point, our thinking shifted, and we started watching therapy to identify what they were doing similarly. As a result, we discovered that all solution focused therapists were doing the same three things in each session.

First, these master clinicians started the conversation by obtaining a desired outcome from the client. The clinicians weren't focusing on a goal or a problem but instead what the client's "best hopes" were—what that person hoped to achieve by coming to therapy.

Second, their sessions included some level of a description, meaning they used solution focused questions to engage the client in a description of the presence of their best hopes. This is where the variance happened among the different sessions, because there are multiple ways to co-construct a description.

Third, they ended their sessions in a way that maintained and honored the client's autonomy. They were careful not to rob clients of being the key contributors of their own change.

All the understanding of SFBT grows from these three things. This is an approach based on a desired outcome; the action you, as a clinician, do is called a description; and in your closing you end the session in a way that has an impact on the client that is likely to lead to more change.

This three-step process (which you'll find on the bar that runs down the left side of the diamond, shown in the image in the next section) might seem simple at a glance, but it took us a long time to figure out that these were the consistent steps that all brilliant solution focused professionals were utilizing in their sessions.

Before we created the diamond, our field had some pretty heated debates about which therapist was doing SFBT correctly, and what we discovered is that they all were practicing it correctly. They were all implementing the same three things in their sessions—a desired outcome, a description, and a closing. That's the language of SFBT. That's the recipe. If you violate that recipe, you're not practicing SFBT.

After we were able to identify the framework of a session in this three-step process, we shifted our focus. Now that we knew *what* solution focused professionals were doing, we then wanted to figure out *how* they were doing it. That led us to create the diamond model.

The Elements of the Diamond Model

Elliott recently saw a client who is a medical doctor, and she conveyed to him in a few words how overwhelmed she felt by the demands of her job. Most psychotherapists would have asked her, "What brought you into therapy?" She would have talked about her lack of sleep and the stress of her job. Instead, as an SFBT therapist, Elliott asked, "What are your best hopes from our talking today?" In other words, he asked what she hoped would be different in her life as a consequence of coming to therapy. She answered, "I want to be more like myself."

The reason SFBT is so interesting is that her answer had nothing to do with the stress of her job, which was the trigger for her coming to therapy. Rather, it had to do with the outcome she wanted—and that desired outcome became the focus of the session.

We've already introduced you to the sidebar of the diamond—the three-step process that includes a desired outcome, a description, and a closing. Now we'll explain the rest of the model.

◆ Important Diamond Definitions ◆

Desired outcome (best hopes): The transformation the client is pursuing in therapy. The best-hopes question can be used to begin the conversation with clients about said transformation.

Description: The detailed explanation of the transformation/desired outcome being present in the client's life.

Closing: How an SFBT session is wrapped up. Typically the focus of this part of the conversation is to ensure that the description from earlier in the conversation is not undone.

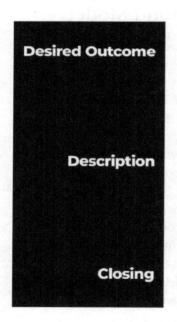

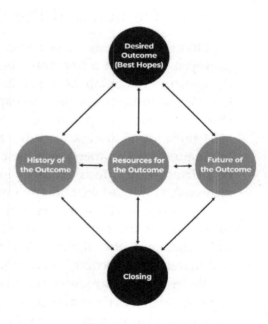

©2021 Elliott Connie & Adam Froerer

The bar on the left shows the three-step process. The diamond-shaped flowchart shows the possible variations in the three-step process.

The bar on the left shows the overall steps of the session. It is like the 10,000-foot view of the approach, whereas the diamond itself is the 10-foot view of the approach. The *desired outcome*, in the top circle of the diamond, runs parallel to its counterpart in the left column. Likewise, the bottom circle, *closing*, runs parallel to its counterpart on the sidebar. Desired outcome and closing are the two unchanging steps in the three-step process of an SFBT session. Where the variance happens is in the *description*, which is represented by the middle row of circles in the diamond (from left to right): *history of the outcome, resource talk,* and *preferred future.* These choices of description pathways are where the diamond gets really interesting.

◆ Special Note about Description Pathways ◆

We use the term *description pathway* to illustrate that each clinician might progress through the diamond in their own unique way. If you think about the diamond like a map, it shows several possible avenues of reaching the same destination. Each clinician will mix their own personal style with the needs and language of the client to determine how to progress through a session. For simplicity we have called the possible progressions *pathways*. There is no right or wrong pathway for a given SFBT session.

History of the outcome is when clients describe the times their desired outcome has shown up in the past and played a role in their life.

Resource talk is when clients describe the strengths, qualities, characteristics, and skills they have that can help them achieve their desired outcome.

Preferred future is when clients describe how their desired outcome will show up in the future, most commonly starting tomorrow.

As we developed this part of the diamond, we considered how to best teach the framework of a session while accounting for the variances within the description. At this point, we had only diagrammed the sidebar and top and bottom circles of the diamond. We didn't know what would go in the middle. Every therapist was doing that part differently. In order to make sense of it all, we decided to study more sessions conducted by master clinicians.

We discovered there are therapists—such as Chris Iveson—who will shift the conversation from the desired outcome to the preferred future. He might ask, "Suppose you woke up tomorrow morning and you were happy?" That's the miracle question, which is a preferred-future question.

There are also therapists—such as Peter Szabo—who will shift the conversation from the desired outcome to discuss the past. He might ask, "Can you tell me about a time that you've been happy in the past?" That's a history-of-the-outcome question.

There are also therapists—such as Evan George—who will shift the conversation from the desired outcome to discuss the client's resources. He might ask, "What might you say that could tip you off that you could possibly achieve that?" That's a resource-talk question.

All of these therapists are practicing SFBT. They are all doing descriptions; they're just choosing different pathways to do so, and that's okay.

After years of analysis, this was our lightbulb moment: there is no one right way to do a description. As long as you are talking about the presence of the desired outcome, you are doing a description.

Furthermore, you can choose to do more than one kind of description in a session. You can even go back to discuss the desired outcome again after spending time doing a description. After all, you're never really done with the desired outcome.

Clients will often say things that amend the first desired outcome they establish. Once you're in the description, you may bounce back to the desired outcome, then back to another description. Even in closing, clients may say something that causes you to backtrack to a previous step. The two-headed arrows in the diamond represent these endless pathway choices.

We've found that all the masters of SFBT have a signature pathway that takes them from desired outcome to closing. Here are just a few:

- **Chris Iveson**: desired outcome → preferred future → closing

- **Harvey Ratner**: desired outcome → scaling* → preferred future → scaling* → closing

- **Evan George**: desired outcome → resource talk → preferred future → scaling* → closing

- **Peter Szabo**: desired outcome → resource talk → history of the outcome → resource talk → closing

- **Steve de Shazer and Insoo Kim Berg**: desired outcome → resource talk → preferred future → scaling* → closing

- **Elliott Connie**: desired outcome → resource talk → preferred future → closing

Scaling was included in our first version of the diamond, but we have come to view it as a tool rather than a pathway, and we'll discuss it more in a later chapter.

In creating the diamond, we wanted to identify a process in which therapists understand that it doesn't matter what variants they choose from within the description pathway, because the masters of this approach were all doing that part of a session differently.

Once we included the description choices in our diagram, our model was complete. Elliott was conducting a training in Chelmsford, England, when he drew the model on a whiteboard for the first time. Someone in the audience commented, "That looks like a diamond," and the name stuck. We've been calling it the diamond since.

The final point of the diamond, closing (the bottom circle), involves ending your session in a way that maintains client autonomy. If you turn into a feedback machine, your clients will feel like you've been assessing them the entire time, which removes their autonomy. Likewise, if you turn into a suggestion robot, that also removes their autonomy.

When you're using SFBT, you have to trust in your clients' ability to achieve change. That means you have to give them the freedom to choose it. Your job is to create an ideal environment. Their job is to utilize that environment and turn it into action.

Keep the closing simple. Simply thank your clients for talking with you, then say something unobtrusive like, "I look forward to seeing what you do." That way your clients can leave to make their own choices about what they'll accomplish with what they have gained from therapy.

The diamond is a flowchart of instructions that will lead you through every part of a session. We'll discuss each component in greater detail in the next few chapters. Together, they comprise the five skills you need to master in order to do solution focused brief therapy well.

We're passionate about this process. The diamond has completely transformed the way we teach SFBT and the way we practice it. We can't wait for you to reap its benefits as well!

From Exceptions to Instances to History of the Outcome

A Closer Look with Adam

Some of the terms Elliott and I use for description pathways originated from Chris Iveson's art gallery metaphor, but you may have noticed the gallery didn't include the history of the outcome.

History of the outcome is a term we coined, and it evolved from what Steve de Shazer and Insoo Kim Berg called exceptions, and what the team at BRIEF in the U.K. later called instances (which we discuss in more detail in Chapter 17, History of the Outcome).

According to Steve and Insoo, exceptions were times in the past when the client's problem wasn't a problem, or times when the problem wasn't as bad. Later at BRIEF, Chris Iveson, Harvey

Ratner, and Evan George were also helping their clients identify exceptions, until they realized that even by talking about exceptions, they were keeping the problem present in a session and therefore inadvertently making the SFBT approach problem-oriented.

The BRIEF team started changing their language and talked instead about instances, meaning times when a client's best hopes were present in the past, even if just by a small occurrence.

Until Elliott and I came along, that's how a client's past had been attended to in SFBT therapy sessions—for Steve and Insoo, through exceptions; and for BRIEF, through instances.

Our term, history of the outcome, grew from instances but also expanded upon it. For example, we realized that we could ask the same kinds of questions in regard to the past in history of the outcome that we do about the future in preferred future.

Preferred Future	History of the Outcome
"Suppose you woke up tomorrow and your best hope was present, what's the very first thing you would notice?"	"When your best hope was present in the past, what did you first notice?"
"Who else would notice?"	"Who else noticed?"
"What would they notice about you?"	"What did they notice about you?"
"What difference would it make in your life?"	"What difference did it make in your life?"

In addition to that, history of the outcome also incorporates what no one else in our field had been talking about, which is what we call legacy questions, which we also discuss in Chapter 17.

Legacy questions are set up by resource-talk questions that refer to the past, such as, "What is it about you that made that best hope possible before?"

Clients will often name some kind of a characteristic about themselves, like, "I guess it's my determination."

From there, the legacy questions can be asked, such as, "Who did you learn that from?"

Clients will usually mention someone really important to them.

If I were to ask Elliott the legacy question above, he would most likely answer, "From my grandmother. She told me she believed in me. She encouraged me to get as much education as possible."

Looking at the client's resources from that viewpoint, it's the legacy that makes the best hopes possible. You can pull forward in the client's timeline and ask, "If your grandmother saw that determination still present in you, what difference would it make to her?"

You can also ask, "If you were able to pass that legacy on to someone else, what difference would it make to you and that person?"

Once you recognize all the possibilities within history of the outcome, you can see how false the criticism is that SFBT is only a future-focused approach. In reality, it's a detail-oriented approach and a difference-oriented approach that takes into consideration the client's past, present, and future in its focus on the desired outcome.

Learning Versus Mastery

Diving Deep with Elliott

I once conducted therapy with a Food Network chef. At the end of our session, we chatted for a bit, and I said to him, "I really like to cook, but I'm not as good as you are. I wish I was as talented."

He smiled and said, "Do you want to know why I'm a better chef than most people?"

I leaned forward, eager to hear his answer. "Yes, I do!"

I thought he was going to share some trick of the trade, like the secret to boiling pasta just right. Instead, he surprised me by saying, "I'm willing to burn more things and not give up. I'm willing to practice the basics even to this day."

Those words still resonate with me. If you're willing to continue practicing the basics and not give up, you become a master.

One of the common but erroneous ways of thinking in the field of psychotherapy is that once you've learned a particular skill, you no longer need to practice it. You can move on to something else. But we don't want you to merely learn SFBT; we want you to become masters of language in sessions with your clients. And mastery requires consistent practice so the edge of your knife can always stay sharp.

There's no way to anticipate what will happen in a session until your clients answer your questions. You won't know the pathway you're going to take on the diamond before they walk into your office. You may know how you'll begin a session (by asking about their best hopes), but after that, the pathway you take is absolutely dependent upon what each client answers.

Becoming a master of language also means you'll become a master at listening. You'll master picking up words from your clients that are consistent with an accurate description of the presence of their desired outcome.

Even years ago when I had just started learning the SFBT approach and wasn't very good yet, I knew what I had to do in order to get good. I needed to practice listening differently, and that involved conveying to my clients that I was not only listening to them but also listening with care.

Don't go into a session with a preconceived notion that you need to impose what you think will be useful on your clients. Instead, co-construct with them what they think will be useful.

The one caveat I'll add is that personality styles do matter. Does Evan George go into every therapy session knowing he's going to follow a predetermined pathway? No. But his inquisitive personality tends to draw him toward his signature pathway of resource talk before he explores other description options.

Becoming a master of SFBT is a combination of honoring who you are as a person while utilizing your client's words, and that blend informs how you develop questions and choose pathways in a session.

You may enjoy one type of description more than another, but it's important to master all of them because you never know when you'll have to venture into a different one.

For example, there are times that I might follow the same pathway on the diamond that Chris Iveson does. There are times that the client says something that makes me intrigued about the history of the outcome. But the most time-worn pathway for me is desired outcome, resource talk, preferred future, and closing.

Going back to the chef analogy, expert chefs are experts of the skill of cooking, and with that skill of cooking, they can improvise within their expertise when unexpected circumstances arise, such as missing ingredients or less time to work with than they thought they'd be given.

The same applies for SFBT therapists. They get good at *all* the skills so they can hone their expertise in just the right way.

Without knowing all the skills, you can't improvise. And you never know what skills you'll have to draw upon.

Don't get discouraged if you try asking the questions we teach in this approach and they don't go as smoothly as you planned. Sometimes therapists give up too soon and say, "SFBT doesn't work." But just like with learning any other skill in life, the more you practice, the better you'll get at it.

Think about when you first rode a bike without training wheels. You probably crashed more than once. But if you had decided that riding a bike was dangerous and you never got on one again, you would have never truly experienced the exhilaration of riding a bike.

As you learn SFBT, don't get caught up in parroting our example questions word for word. Learning them verbatim isn't what we want you to focus on. Instead, we want you to learn our process. We want you to turn into question builders, not just question askers, because questions are integral in each part of the diamond.

In the following chapters, we'll walk you through those parts. We'll teach you the skills necessary to conduct a session in a way that is authentic to you and transformative to your clients. Soon you'll become an expert who can improvise and adapt and become truly confident in your work.

Chapter 11

Desired Outcome

The Top Point of the Diamond

Take the Stance That
Your Client Can Achieve Change

Diving Deep with Elliott

A mom recently brought her teenager, Alexis (name changed), to see me for therapy. Alexis had a serious health concern that she'd dealt with all her life, but when she turned 16, she was tired of managing her illness and stopped taking her medications. Her doctors and mom had been trying to get her to be med-compliant, but Alexis didn't care. Even when they told her she was putting her life at risk by not taking her medicine, that didn't change her attitude and actions.

When I met Alexis, I could have taken the position that she was a difficult teenager who wasn't following the rules, but instead I took the stance of trusting her capability to achieve change. I also focused on what my job entails, which boils down to two things: asking my client what she's hoping to achieve, then asking questions to help that outcome become more likely than not.

I began doing just that when I asked, "What is it you're hoping to achieve from talking with me today, Alexis?"

She crossed her arms. "I don't know. I don't want to be here."

I nodded with understanding. "Since you are here and we're going to have a chat, what do you hope the outcome will be in your life?"

She narrowed her eyes. "I doubt you can help with what I want to be."

"I might not be able to," I replied. "But if you could share it with me, I'd love to hear it."

She nibbled on her lip for a moment before answering, "I'd love to be a college cheerleader."

Now I could have stopped believing in Alexis right then. I didn't know whether she could cheer, or what level of talent college cheerleading required. After all, I've never been a college cheerleader. But I did know that in order to become a college cheerleader, Alexis would have to become a college student, and in order to become a college student, she would have to be alive.

"What do you find exciting about being a college cheerleader?" I asked, trying to find a foundation of her best hopes.

She uncrossed her arms. "Well, they're really popular and have lots of friends." She went on to talk more about the great social life she dreamed of having one day.

As I listened through what she was telling me, I understood that what she wanted most in life was to be accepted and treated as though she were a "normal" teenager. Her health issues and medications made her feel less than normal, which for a teenage girl had to be super challenging.

"What would you notice about yourself if you woke up tomorrow and found yourself on a path that would help make what you want in life become more likely?"

She took a deep breath. "I'd have to take my medicine."

"And how would you remember that taking your medicine was a part of creating this future that you're so hopeful about?"

She looked out the window, deep in thought. "Well, when I think about it, I want to take my medicine because I want that future to happen."

I saw Alexis three times in total. After our last session, her mom visited with me briefly over Zoom. "What have you done?" she asked, astonished. "Alexis and I don't argue about her taking her medicine anymore. She has been 100 percent medically compliant for three months now. And when I took her to see her doctor a week ago, her lab work showed optimal levels for her condition. What have you done?"

The answer was simple. I took the stance before Alexis even walked into my office—the stance I hold on to throughout every moment of every session—that Alexis wasn't difficult, resistant, or noncompliant. That stance was the unshakeable belief that she could change.

The Critical Difference
between a Goal and an Outcome

Have you ever been told that solution focused brief therapy is a goal-oriented approach to psychotherapy? People continue to claim this, but the masters of the approach intentionally use the word *outcome* now instead of *goal* (as in goal-oriented) because the two words are dynamically different.

One important distinction between goals and outcomes is how people go about them. For example, when people try to achieve goals, they usually resort to problem-solving. They think that an obstacle must be in their way, so they brainstorm how to get past it and deliberate on options regarding how to obtain their goal.

If they try the best option they come up with and don't succeed, their confidence takes a hit. Their desire to persevere plummets. They might move on to another option, or they might give up altogether.

Trying to achieve a desired outcome is vastly different from achieving a goal because *outcome* implies that endless possibilities exist. How to get there isn't relevant in an SFBT session. When you *are*, there is the focus. Describing the presence of the outcome and what difference it would make are what drive lasting determination and change.

If you merely focus on how to get there, then your questions get stuck in the rut of "What could you do?" For example, "What could you do to get your partner to like you better?" or "What could you do to control your tongue and not argue so much?"

In contrast, when you focus on the outcome already being present, you don't have to worry about how to get there. You're free to ask questions like, "When you feel peaceful, what do you notice that is different?"

In some sense, a goal can be thought of as a stepping stone in obtaining a desired outcome, or at least the mechanism to help you figure that out.

When asked the best-hopes question, clients usually first answer by declaring a goal or a strategy. They might say something like, "I want my partner to stop sleeping around." That statement explains *what* your client wants, but you need to think beyond that and ask additional questions that illuminate *why* your client wants it.

Motivational speakers bring up this topic frequently. "You've got to know your *why*," they say. That's the same thing we're trying to nuance in distinguishing goals from outcomes. As a therapist, you need to essentially ask your clients, "If that's your goal, why is it your goal?" We don't typically use the word *why* overtly, but we get at the same thing by asking questions such as, "What difference would achieving that make to you?" When you understand the difference it will make to your clients, you are much more likely to understand their *why*.

Once you ask about the *why*, your clients will delve deeper. "We would fall in love again," they might answer, which is a more transformative response than, "I want my partner to stop sleeping around." Their partner not sleeping around is only part of what your client really wants. Your client being in love again is a more meaningful outcome—a more meaningful transformation.

Asking questions about difference is a great way to help your client establish that meaningful outcome at the beginning of a session. That's how solution focused therapists ask their clients about their *why*.

In another scenario, let's say your client is a father who declares that he wants to lose 20 pounds. "What difference would it make if you lost twenty pounds?" you ask him. His answer—the *why*—is that his doctor told him that if he doesn't lose weight, he might not live much longer due to an increased heart risk. This concerns him because he loves his young daughter, and he wants to be around for several more years so he can attend her high school graduation.

By knowing the why, you can now home in on what motivates this father. Statistically speaking, one of the reasons why people fail to lose weight is because they focus on the number of pounds they want to shed rather than *why* they want to shed them.

Remember, the goal is what the client wants—in this case, pounds shed—but the outcome is what drives that person to take action about it. If all the father focuses on is "I want to lose twenty pounds," he'll eventually lose discipline and abandon his pursuit.

Going back to Chris Iveson as the developer of the best-hopes question, despite the fact that he told Elliott he had given up on teaching about best hopes, he actually regrouped and started teaching the subject again—with our push to do so. One important observation that Chris has made regarding desired outcomes is how to identify when you've established a really good one—and that's when the client finally answers the best-hopes question by naming an internal state.

So what is the internal state that the father wants to achieve by losing 20 pounds so he can live long enough to attend his daughter's high school graduation? It's love. It's satisfaction in seeing all the years of his parenting finally pay off.

SFBT is never about the 20 pounds or the partner who should stop sleeping around or whatever your clients label as their problem. Instead it's about things such as familial love and satisfaction, falling in love again, and feeling peace and acceptance. It's those internal states that really matter.

You ask the best-hopes question to be introduced to your clients' hearts, and you need to try to speak to their hearts as much as possible throughout the rest of the session. You do that by using the specific language they have given you to describe what's in their hearts.

Again, *listen through* to what your clients are really saying. Help them say it for themselves. Move beyond their surface-level problems and dig deeper to uncover what they're truly hoping to achieve in their lives.

Making "Impossible" Outcomes Linguistically Possible

Clients often talk about themselves or their problems in a way that brings about doubt for themselves—and if you're not careful, for you. But your job is to maintain the very stubborn belief that your clients are capable of change, no matter what they say about themselves or their problems. Solution focused questions don't live in the desert of doubt; they live in the forest of hope.

If a client says she wants her deceased husband to be alive again, it's your job as a therapist to take that seemingly impossible desired outcome and make it linguistically possible. This means that you take the client completely seriously. You linguistically make it possible by saying something like, "And if your husband was alive again, what difference would that make to you?" This gives the client the opportunity to say something like, "I would be happy again." Now you have moved into a territory of possibility; happiness can be present. We can ask a question like, "And if you found yourself feeling happy in the same way that you might if your husband were to be alive again, what would be the first thing that would let you know that this kind of happiness was back in your life?" Notice the linguistic mastery that is necessary to move the conversation to happiness rather than being founded upon a resurrected husband. It is the job of the therapist to take the client seriously *and* linguistically co-construct a possible desired outcome.

If another client answers your best-hopes question by replying, "I don't know. I've been depressed my whole life," you might panic and think, *If they've been depressed their whole life, how am I going to do something about it?*

Once doubt creeps into your mind, you are no longer operating from a position of hope, and as a solution focused therapist, you need to hold on to hope at all costs. You can learn how to do that. Holding on to hope is a skill you can develop like any other.

One of Elliott's clients was a woman named Laura (name changed), who has a nonverbal son with a severe brain injury. When Elliott asked Laura the best-hopes question, she answered, "I want to hear my son call me *Mom*."

Upon hearing that, part of Elliott automatically thought, *Wow, that's difficult*. It's emotional. It drew him in. But the other part of him understood that his job is to make Laura's outcome linguistically possible, meaning he needed to engage her in a conversation in which she has what she wants. Whether her son will ever be able to talk is not related to his job, and in some sense, none of his business.

Elliott said to Laura, "Gosh, I don't know how this could happen or if it's even possible, but if somehow after our talking today, your son could start calling you *Mom*, what difference would that make to you?"

"Oh, that would be wonderful because I've been stuck on wanting this for so long," she said. "Things would finally be the way they're supposed to be."

"And when you're finally feeling that things are the way they should be, instead of being stuck on whether or not your son can call you *Mom*, what would you be thinking about instead?"

"I guess I would feel like I was a normal mom."

Did you notice that, even though Laura said what she wants is for her son to call her *Mom*, what she actually wants is to be a normal mom? In SFBT, you need to delve deeper from the client's stated outcome to the client's actualized outcome. This idea expands upon the concept of goals versus outcomes.

A stated outcome is one that could create doubt, but an actualized outcome is one that creates hope. And an actualized outcome means more than just a realistic outcome. That's why we use the word *actualized* rather than *actual* to define it.

Laura's stated outcome was, "I want my son to call me *Mom*," but the actualization of that—the result of that, if it were to happen—is that Laura would feel like a normal mom. Notice that the actualized outcome is still using the client's language.

If Elliott were a magician, he could snap his fingers and make Laura's son call her *Mom*, but that's not truly what she wants. She wants what would happen next, which is the actualization of it, meaning that when her son says *Mom*, she would get a warm and fuzzy feeling that she identifies as "feeling like a normal mom."

Again, it's helpful to think of the desired outcome (or actualized outcome) as an internal state that the client can control. Laura has no control over whether her son can call her *Mom*, but she does have control over her own experience, so that's what the session should focus on.

Once you establish an actualized outcome—in Laura's case, "to feel like a normal mom"—you can shift to the description portion of the diamond and co-construct the presence of the outcome with your client. More will be mentioned about these pathways in chapters to come.

The Stance of Autonomy
Begins with Best Hopes

A Closer Look with Adam

Elliott and I discuss autonomy the most when we're teaching about closing a session—the end point of the diamond. However, honoring the client's autonomy isn't a discipline to be saved for only closing time. It actually begins at the start of a session. Your very first question to the client is, "What are your best hopes?"

One of the presuppositions embedded in that question is often overlooked. The therapist is asking the client, "What are your best hopes?" In other words, "What do you want?" Sometimes clients will answer by sharing what their teacher or spouse or probation officer wants them to do. You need to steer them back on track by asking, "But what are your best hopes?"

Keep in mind that you need to respect what they want as well. If your client declares something big and grand like, "I want to be a millionaire," don't reply, "Hmm, can you be more realistic? What if you just considered the first step you'd need to take in order to become a millionaire?"

When you argue with what your clients want, or when you offer suggestions, you remove their autonomy, which removes their ownership of creating change.

Instead, if you start a session with autonomy and hold on to it by building an entire conversation around what your clients want, then when you get to the end of a session, it should be easy to allow them to choose what they want to do with what they've gained from therapy, rather than assigning them a task or homework.

Build the expectation of autonomy from the moment your clients walk into your office, and do everything you can throughout the session to protect it. This is hugely important when you're working with couples and families. Don't allow any individual to violate the autonomy of another person in your office. Don't take sides. Don't buy into the talk that the burden to change only falls on one person instead of everyone present. It's your job to safeguard each person's autonomy. We'll share some examples of how to do that in the next chapter.

Shifting from Outcomes to Transformations

Diving Deep with Elliott

It may be helpful for you to think of desired outcomes as desired transformations. The latter term is clearer because clients aren't really coming to therapy for an outcome; they're coming to transform. Clients hire you because they don't like who they are today, and they want you to help them transform into someone that they'd like to be tomorrow. They're caterpillars, and they want to become butterflies.

Solution focused brief therapy is a change-oriented approach. You're looking for difference, and the word *transformation* captures that. It also helps you focus on whom the client wants to be when you're working to establish a meaningful best-hopes answer.

For example, if you had conducted therapy with 19-year-old Elliott, you would have been talking to a very anxious, depressed, and suicidal person. My life was in complete flux. If you had asked me then, "What are your best hopes from our talking?" I would have wanted you to be thinking, *Who do you want to be, Elliott?*

You would have had to work hard to get a best-hopes answer from me because I was in such dire straits back then. I probably wouldn't have told you, "I want to be happy." I probably would have said, "I don't even know how to answer that question. Things are so dark and difficult right now."

Another important word to keep in mind is *version*, because the clients you meet with are not who they want to be yet. This is just a version of them. I wouldn't have wanted you to think of 19-year-old me as a depressed, anxious, and suicidal person. I would have wanted you to think this was only a version of me.

The clients who come into your office are going to be the addicted version of themselves, the depressed version, the anxious version, the "not following their parents' rules" version, whatever the case may be. If you're working with a couple, they might come in as the unhappy version of that couple.

If you accept the label of "we're unhappy," then it's really hard for you to believe *in* your clients and therefore do your job well. But if you can adjust your mindset to believe that who is before you is just an unhappy version, then you can also believe that a happy version is buried underneath whatever challenges this couple or this person is currently having.

It's up to you to co-construct with your clients what transformation they're looking for, and it's up to your clients to figure out how to bring about that transformation into their lives. Sometimes that means changing back into a version they have been before.

When a client tells me, "I want to be happy," I don't even have to ask, "Have you ever been happy?" I can simply presuppose that this client has experienced happiness before. "When in your life do you remember being the most happy?" I can ask, and I can do so with extraordinary confidence. Why? No matter how difficult life has been, every person has experienced some measure of happiness in the past. Therefore every person is also capable of achieving *new* happiness.

Whenever people say they want something, they're also admitting they've tasted it before. That's the way the brain works. You can't crave something you've never sampled.

So remember to believe in your clients. Don't disrespect them by thinking they haven't experienced any moments of happiness before, regardless of how challenging their story is or has been.

Conditional Presuppositions

A Closer Look with Adam

Presuppositions are deeply connected with desired outcomes, and when presuppositions are contingent upon those desired outcomes, they help clients achieve lasting change in a rapid amount of time.

Conditional presuppositions are instances when the therapist asks a question with the presupposition that a specific condition is in place for the client (Froerer et al.).

For example, if the client's best hope is to be happy, the therapist could apply a conditional presupposition by asking, "If you woke up tomorrow and felt happy, what is the first thing you would notice?" The question is contingent upon that specific condition being in place.

A conditional presupposition has the pattern of "If your best hope is present"—that's the condition—"how does that change things?"

In the same vein, you can ask:

"Who's going to notice?"

"What are they going to notice?"

"How are they going to notice?"

"What difference does it make to you that they notice?"

All of those questions are based on the client's best hopes being present.

Over the decades that SFBT has been practiced, clients are attending therapy for shorter and shorter amounts of time. Why? Because SFBT therapists are spending more and more of that time essentially telling them, "Focus on your best hopes."

"If your best hope is present, what difference would that make?"

"What transformation would happen?"

"If your transformation happens, what would you notice?"

"If that transformation happens, how would your life be different?"

When you presuppose *and* build in the condition that your clients' best hopes are present, they will transform remarkably quickly. And isn't that what any good therapist wants—to help their clients succeed?

That's why it's so critical to establish a solid and meaningful best-hopes answer from each client you work with, then ask every follow-up question as if it's connected to those best hopes.

Presuppose that your clients' best hopes completely encompass their entire lives.

Recognizing When to
Move Forward in the Diamond

Therapists are sometimes unsure when to move forward in the diamond from desired outcome to the various description pathways. This uncertainty usually happens when therapists are working with clients who don't divulge emotional information as quickly as others, and so it takes those clients longer to articulate a meaningful best-hopes answer.

As previously discussed, one of the indicators that your client has given a meaningful best-hopes answer is that they have named an internal state. But sometimes they don't need to get all the way to the internal state in the desired-outcome portion of the diamond; sometimes just being close to naming it is enough for you to expand upon as you move forward to a description.

Another indicator for knowing when to shift from desired outcome to a description is identifying something from your clients' answers that you can continue to ask questions about in a passionate way. We're guessing that most people would be much more interested in hearing the answers to questions about "being the mom I'm supposed to be" more than they would be interested in hearing details about what it would take to "lose twenty-five pounds." Often clients will begin by telling us their desired outcome is to lose 25 pounds. When we ask what difference it would make for them to lose 25 pounds, we often hear something much more meaningful, such as "being the parent I'm supposed to be." We wouldn't be passionate about a weight-loss description, but we could get very passionate with purposeful-parent descriptions. If you can feel passionate about the questions you ask, your clients can feel passionate about the answers they give you. This co-construction will feel energizing rather than burdensome for both you and your client. Keep persevering when trying to establish a best-hopes answer until you sense that you've found the hook for the rest of the conversation—the thing that gets you excited.

Elliott likes to use the term *currency* when talking about this concept. What's the client's currency? What really motivates that person? What is their "why" for doing what they do when they are behaving consistent with what is most meaningful to them? What is it that the client values most? If we go back to the example of the mom being the kind of mom she is supposed to be and ask that mom simply to get up at 4 A.M. to work out, she would likely say, "No way!" However, if we told her that if she woke up at 4 A.M. and worked out, her children would be guaranteed to be happy every day, she would very likely get up each morning at 4 A.M. Her kids are her currency. She is at her best when she remembers that her kids are important to her.

The third indicator for establishing a meaningful best-hopes answer is that it is broad enough for you to continue asking questions about it for 45 minutes. You don't want to build a session around something narrow, such as losing 25 pounds, because there is a finite number of strategies to accomplish this goal. On the other hand, the parent-they-are-supposed-to-be could be described quite differently when the parent is at home, when at the children's school, by their partner, through the eyes of the children, etc. When we choose to co-construct a broad outcome, the number of questions we can build on is limitless.

What Is a Good-Enough Best Hopes?

♦ You have a name for the best hopes (e.g., hope, confidence, peace, or happiness).

♦ You are excited about asking more detailed questions about the named best hopes.

♦ The desired outcome is about a *transformation* of the client.

♦ Something inside of the client changes (i.e., they have more hope).

♦ Something outside the client changes because the client changes (e.g., their family is getting along better).

♦ The desired outcome is based on the client's currency (a.k.a., what is most meaningful to them).

♦ You feel confident that you can ask questions about this transformation for the bulk of the session.

Remember that bar on the left side of the diamond? It lists the three things you have to do in a therapy session: obtain a desired outcome, get a description, and end with a closing.

Closing takes about two minutes. So from the time you obtain a desired outcome until the two minutes you reserve for closing, the only other thing you're going to be doing in a session is getting a description.

Find a best-hopes answer that motivates you and your client to have a rich and engaging therapy session.

When Clients Get Stuck Answering, "I Don't Know"

At the beginning of a session, your clients will often answer the best-hopes question by saying, "I don't know" or "I haven't thought of that before." That's okay. That's a marker that they are creating a new reality in real time through their language.

One of our colleagues, Dr. Mark McKergow, refers to this process as "brain stretching" because it requires a great deal of concentration and effort. Through the questions you ask, you are stretching your clients' thinking and experience. You are watching them transform before your eyes.

So pat yourself on the back when your clients answer, "I don't know." That answer is a clue that you're on the right track. Solution focused conversations should not be easy. Don't give up, and don't let your clients off the hook when they get stuck answering, "I don't know."

This is the prime example of not believing your client but believing in your client. Trust that they do know the answer and that you can help them find it with respectful persistence.

You do this by becoming a master of listening. Remember what they say, take their language, and use it to formulate your next question. If they answer, "I don't know," you can take that language and reply, "Suppose you took a minute and thought about it and came up with something that you *did* know. How would you answer then?"

Let's say they divulge a bit more by saying, "I still don't know. I just don't feel confident in any answer," you could take that language and reply, "If I had asked you this question at the time you were the most confident in an answer, what would you have said then?"

Every time you ask a new question, clients usually give a little more of an answer than just "I don't know," and you can use that new language to keep persisting with additional questions until they break the cycle.

The interesting thing is, once the cycle is broken, clients rarely revert back to answering, "I don't know." This is likely because they are beginning to catch the vision of the best hopes—they're starting to actually allow themselves to believe that the transformation they desire could be present in their lives. It might also be that they finally trust you enough to tell you something really personal to them, perhaps something they haven't ever shared with anyone else.

If your clients' answers aren't getting clearer and you seem to be going in circles, then use their language in a way that minimizes their options. Consider the following scenario:

You: What are your best hopes from talking to me?

Client: I don't know. I just want to feel happy.

You: What difference would it make for you to feel happy?

Client: Well, I guess I'd feel good inside.

You: If you felt good inside, what impact would that have on you?

Client: I already said—it would make me feel happy.

You can see how that would quickly turn into a loop. One of the things you can do is anticipate the loop and build that loop into your next question in a way that forces a different answer.

You could ask, "If you felt happy and also felt good inside, what would be the first thing that would let you know that both of those things existed at the same time?"

Build in the answers you've already been given, using your clients' language to formulate a question that anticipates the loop. Doing so minimizes their options. It becomes harder for them to put you off or answer vaguely. Figuratively but respectfully, you have backed them into a corner until they can finally "brain stretch" enough to give you a meaningful answer.

Again, don't give up. At the heart of SFBT is care and love. We care about our clients, and we don't give up on people that we care about. Keep persisting for no other reason than if you stop persisting that demonstrates the absence of care.

Additionally, don't overintellectualize your job. Don't get caught up in implementing the perfect technique to push past the "I don't knows" or any roadblock. Remember, SFBT is heart work. Caring about your clients is where the ability to persist comes from. It's what should motivate you rather than any theory.

Decide to "out-care" any difficulty you encounter in a session. Focus on holding on to the stubborn belief that your clients can achieve change. They need to know they're capable, even if they're struggling. Giving up on a question is giving up on your clients, and you can't allow that to happen.

Remember that SFBT is not client-led; it's outcome-led. And if you care about your clients, you're going to help them achieve their outcomes. That begins by asking however many questions are necessary in establishing a meaningful desired outcome—a meaningful best hope.

Keep persisting and believing because solution focused brief therapy happens on the other side of that answer for your clients.

How to Respond to Content

Sometimes clients like to give you content when you try to establish their best hopes. For example, a client may tell you, "I think my boyfriend is cheating on me. He's gone a lot at night."

That's content, and obtaining content doesn't necessarily fall within the bounds of your job. If your client gives you content, then you need to work to place it within the realm of your job.

If you're in the best-hopes portion of the session, bring the conversation back to establishing a desired outcome. You can reply to your client's content with something like, "If your boyfriend is cheating on you, what do you think would be a useful thing for us to do during this session?" or "If you're unsure if your boyfriend is cheating on you, what do we need to do here that would be useful to you?" In other words, you're asking, "Given where you are with this uncertainty, how do we utilize this time in a way that's just right for you?"

The content that was presented to you may be difficult for your client, so remember to acknowledge that difficulty, but also remember that the content in and of itself doesn't help you do your job. Don't get distracted or overwhelmed by content. Sometimes when clients throw content in, it's easy to get diverted and think, *Wow, that's such a hard struggle. I need to talk about this content or my client is going to feel hurt or ignored or think I don't care.* But you can acknowledge the content in such a way that still respects the client and moves the session forward.

How to Recognize When You Are Hearing Content

♦ Details shared are about what is currently happening in the client's life rather than what they would like to be happening.

♦ Details provided are related to the problem or the issue that brought the client to therapy.

♦ The details don't add something to the transformation the client is looking for.

♦ The information provides details about what the client doesn't want rather than contributing to what they do want.

In the scenario above, because the client has introduced their boyfriend through content, you might find a useful opportunity to bring him up later in the session. For example, you could say, "Suppose that peace and happiness and joy (the desired outcome) fell into your life, what difference would that make with the way you're interacting with your boyfriend?" However, the boyfriend may or may not be relevant to the session and the scope of your job in the session, so you don't always have to find a way to use content.

You might be wondering what to do with clients who really want to talk about content. Our answer is let them talk about it. Remember, every answer that your clients give is the right answer. All you're there to do is to ask questions that are consistent with your job. Your clients get to answer in whatever way they want to answer. Maintain their autonomy. Don't say, "Nope. We don't talk about what you've brought up here." If you do that, you're essentially telling them they're not autonomous in the conversation.

Instead, listen through the content they give and presuppose the best in them. If a client comes to therapy and says she thinks her boyfriend is cheating on her, listen through that and think, *Wow, this woman must be super strong to come to therapy given what she believes is going on with her partner.*

As you *listen through* your clients' answers, you'll find strength, resources, and resiliency. Use those to build questions with positive presuppositions embedded in them, such as, "Given that you're facing this difficult uncertainty, how are you the kind of person that continues to persevere in life?"

Questions with positive presuppositions recognize your clients' struggles while also conveying your faith in their ability to overcome them.

Do Clients Feel Bombarded by Questions?

People often ask if our clients feel bombarded with questions in solution focused brief therapy. Honestly, they don't. The questions we ask might feel repetitive to a casual observer, but when you're the person having to answer those questions—questions that hit at the heart of what you want most in life—answering requires so much concentration that the last thing you are thinking of is the number of questions you've been asked so far, or if any of those questions are similar.

Questions don't feel the same to clients because clients answer differently each time. They are co-constructing their outcome with you, and with each answer they give, they add additional language to that outcome. The details they describe turn that outcome into their new reality.

What If Clients Want Someone Else to Change?

When clients are asked to answer the best-hopes question, their first few answers might be responses like, "I don't need to change anything about myself. It's other people who need to change so my life can get better." What Elliott does in this situation is he asks, "What difference would it make to you if they actually did change?"

When you ask a "what difference" question, and you add "to you" ("What difference would that make to you?"), the focus automatically shifts to the client instead of other people. It shifts internally instead of externally and helps the client take ownership.

You may have to ask "what difference" questions a few times before your clients finally answer in regard to themselves rather than others. That's when you'll arrive at a best-hopes answer that you can use to co-construct the rest of the session around.

Consider Important People to Your Client

Oftentimes when you're looking for your clients' desired outcome, what you're trying to get at is *purpose*. What would they give everything for?

A key thing you can ask about in order to get to that purpose are the people who are the most important to your clients. In Elliott's case, he would do anything to make his grandmother proud.

Your clients' purpose is often tied to their relationships. When clients are asked, "What difference would that make?" they frequently answer by sharing how important people in their lives will be affected.

From there, it's helpful to ask, "If you can make a difference in their lives, what difference would that make to you?" Now you'll get an answer about the direct impact on your clients, which helps them to bring the focus back inward and to deliver those internal-state answers you're looking for, like being happy, feeling fulfilled, having energy, and living life with a purpose.

Chapter 12

Desired Outcome

Working with Couples

Merging Two Outcomes with Couples

Diving Deep with Elliott

When I started working with couples over 15 years ago, I couldn't find any books on the subject of SFBT with couples, at least any that were written to help therapists.

Stumped on a tenet I knew I would have to face, I called Adam and asked, "When you have two clients in a session, do you discuss two desired outcomes or one?"

"That's a really interesting and important question," he replied, then admitted, "I don't know." Neither of us could think of a time this topic had been addressed by any professional in our field.

As we started digging for an answer, I considered what I *did* know about working with couples. I recalled being taught that the couple's *relationship* is the client, not the people who make up that couple. Consequently, I resolved to establish one desired outcome per couple.

Adam and I started practicing couples therapy following that new rule. We asked each partner what he or she hoped to achieve, and then tied both separate outcomes together. Our sessions were clunky and difficult at first, until I had a lightbulb moment while working with one particular married couple, Chad and Maura (names changed).

Maura began to cry when I asked her what her best hopes were. Reaching for a tissue on my desk, she replied, "All I want is another baby."

As soon as she answered, Chad's face turned rock-hard. "Over my dead body," he said.

I'll never forget sitting across from them, thinking, *What on earth am I going to do?* Despite my panic, I realized this was a prime opportunity to practice what Adam and I had been talking about in regard to merging outcomes.

As sensitively as possible, I said to Maura, "Let's imagine after successful therapy that you and Chad decide that having a baby *is* a good idea. What difference would that make to you?"

She proceeded to tell me how she had been an only child growing up, which was a terrible experience for her, so she'd promised herself to never have just one child like her parents did. "If I could have another baby and give my son a sibling," she said, "I would feel like I was living God's purpose for me as a mom."

In that moment, I realized something important: this woman could be living God's purpose for her as a mom regardless if she had one child or a thousand children. This was not a therapy session about whether she should have another baby. This was a therapy session about the feeling that was behind having another baby.

I asked her another question. "After successful therapy, whether or not you and Chad have another baby, if you definitely felt like you were fulfilling God's purpose for you as a mom, would you be pleased?"

She looked me squarely in the eye and answered, "Yes, I'd be very pleased."

Did you catch how the conversation shifted? We were no longer talking about Maura having another baby; we were discussing the internal state she hoped to achieve as a mom.

I turned to Chad and said, "Let's imagine after successful therapy that you and Maura decide *not* to have another baby. What difference would that make to you?"

He told me about the stress and pressure he was under as the owner of a small company, as well as being the sole provider for his family. He worried about making ends meet right now and in the future. Additionally, he didn't want Maura to suffer through intense infertility treatments again, like she had to when she'd gotten pregnant before. He described watching her go through that as the hardest thing he'd ever seen. "When my wife talks about having another baby, it just freaks me out," he said. "At the end of the day, I just want to be a good provider."

Another lightbulb went off for me. This wasn't a session about whether Chad wanted to have another baby with Maura. This was a session about him feeling secure and wanting to be a good provider, which was connected to his love and concern for his wife.

"After successful therapy, regardless if you and Maura have another baby," I asked him, "if you felt like a good provider, would you be pleased?"

He lifted his downcast eyes. "Yes, I'd be pleased."

I addressed Chad and Maura as a couple now. "Suppose you woke up tomorrow, and Maura, you felt like you were living God's purpose for you as a mom, with or without another baby, and Chad, you felt like you were a good provider, with or without another baby, what would you notice?"

We proceeded to co-construct a description of the presence of feeling like a good mom and the presence of feeling like a good provider. This worked as the one outcome for this couple—one combinable outcome as Adam will explain below. Watching Chad and Maura come alive with hope as they answered my questions felt like genuine magic.

After I worked with them for a few sessions, I didn't hear from them again until a couple of years later when I received an e-mail from Chad. He thanked me for the therapy I'd provided for them and updated me on their lives. He said he'd sold his company and they had moved to another state.

"By the way," he added, "I've attached a picture of me holding my new babies—twin boys. Thank you for your role in helping me grow my family."

The gift of that e-mail reinforced to me the power of language. I hadn't taught Chad and Maura what to do or how to solve their problem. I simply had a conversation that engaged them in an outcome—one combinable outcome since they were a couple—and I trusted that they could achieve it.

If I never help another couple for as long as I live, I'll be satisfied knowing I was influential in helping this couple grow their family.

An Analysis of Couples Therapy

A Closer Look with Adam

As soon as you have more than one client in a session, you have an extra-layered job. When you work with individuals, you're co-constructing an outcome with just one person. But as soon as you introduce a second person, now you have two best-hopes answers. Your job as a therapist is to merge those answers gradually until you can co-construct one desired outcome.

Remember to believe in your clients. That means taking each one of their best-hopes answers seriously, even if those answers are polar opposite. Ask each partner, "If you were to get that outcome, what difference would that make to you?"

In the example Elliott shared above, the difference for Maura was living God's purpose for her as a mom. That's an outcome Chad would also want for her, as opposed to her initial stated goal of wanting another baby. Hearing Maura's deeper answer affects the way Chad views her. Now she isn't being selfish by wanting something he doesn't want, and now she isn't someone who doesn't care about his financial worries for their family; instead, she's someone who is living according to what she sees as God's purpose for her.

Conversely, when Elliott asked Chad what difference his best hopes would make, which Chad answered as being a good provider, Maura also now sees her husband in a new light. Being a good provider is different from "I don't want a baby." Being a good provider impacts Maura positively, because when Chad's a good provider, he's providing for her, taking care of her needs, and helping her in some sense become more in line with who she says God wants her to be.

Each question you ask your clients who come to couples therapy brings their language closer together, which in turn brings them one step closer to merging their desired outcomes and creating a new reality.

Once those outcomes are merged as closely as possible through obtaining their refined best-hopes answers, you can then ask your clients what difference those outcomes would make to them as a couple, just like Elliott did. "If you were to live God's purpose for you," he asked Maura, "and if you were able to be a good provider," he asked Chad, "what difference would that make to you as a couple?"

Do you see how he took their extremely opposing desired outcomes (initially stated as wanting a baby and not wanting a baby) and merged them into one question, one narrative? In doing so, he is now addressing the relationship as his client—a relationship made up of people who respect and value and love one another.

When people can view each other in the best light and realize that what they want is in line with each other, then they can make decisions on their own about what is good for them.

While you're on the quest to obtain a meaningful desired outcome from each partner, try to pull things from each person that can be combined with the other person's contribution. For instance, *friendship* and *peacefulness* are answers that can be easily combined.

At first, Maura's and Chad's answers weren't combinable. "I want a baby" and "I don't want a baby" can't be woven together into the same narrative. Elliott had to dig deeper until he found outcomes that could combine. "Living God's purpose as a mom" and "being a good provider" were combinable answers. They both conveyed doing one's best for the family.

Acknowledge the Environment

In couples therapy, you may work with clients who have extremely opposing answers as to whether they want to remain partners. Perhaps when you ask the best-hopes question, a wife answers that she wants to leave her husband, but he says that he wants her to stay.

To illustrate how you can handle this scenario, imagine you dig deeper by asking what difference it would make for each partner if they got their stated goals (to leave or to stay in the relationship), and they establish the desired outcomes of "pure joy" from the wife and "feeling better" from the husband. Those are outcomes that *can* be woven together, but how can you do so sensitively when the couple first presented such opposing answers about wanting to stay together?

You might say something to the wife like, "Listen, I know it's been hard for you. There's no way to hide the hurt and challenges you've experienced with your husband. I'm not sure if you want to stay in the relationship, but let's say you woke up tomorrow and for whatever reason the pure joy you've been searching for happens. It doesn't wait for your husband to be out of your life. Again, I'm not sure how yet, but the pure joy is just present."

You can then address the husband and add, "Suppose this 'feeling better' emotion that you've been talking about is no longer dependent upon whether your wife stays or goes. For whatever reason, you just woke up tomorrow morning feeling better."

Now addressing them as a couple, you can ask, "What's the very first thing you would notice that would let you know that, while your situation is still difficult and strained, pure joy and feeling better have already arrived?"

Do you see how that last question takes both individuals' answers and turns them into one narrative? There's no need to problem-solve. You don't have to figure out why the wife wants to leave or why the husband wants her to stay. You only have to focus on the constraints of your job as an SFBT therapist: to establish an outcome, even when it's difficult, and co-construct a description about it.

Just because you're not a problem-solver doesn't mean you're a problem-ignorer, however. It's still important to acknowledge the problem by acknowledging the environment and also matching its intensity.

If you act enthusiastic when the couple isn't and exclaim, "Suppose you woke up tomorrow and you were experiencing pure joy and feeling better?" you would sound like a jackass because you wouldn't be acknowledging the environment.

Instead, remember to respect the difficulty and pain that your clients are experiencing. Match their intensity by acknowledging the emotions in the room and use the language your clients have given you.

You can say something to the wife like, "Look, I can see it in your eyes. You're really hurt and strained and angry. But let's say you woke up tomorrow, and you're not sure how it happened, but the pure joy you're seeking just showed up."

You need to also honor the husband's position. You might say, "I know you're hurt and you're struggling, and I'm not sure how yet, but let's imagine that amongst that hurt and struggle, this sense of feeling better just happened, and it was no longer dependent upon what's going on with your wife."

From there, when you go on to ask what both of them would notice if their outcome was present, remember to do so as if you've been listening to their pain.

Acknowledging the environment also means acknowledging that your clients have rational reasons for their best hopes. If the wife wants to leave her husband, you have to trust that there's a good reason for that—a reason she defines as "pure joy." Likewise, there's a valid reason that the husband wants her to stay, which, in his words, is to "feel better."

In shifting to a description pathway, acknowledging the environment also means admitting you have no idea how the outcome will happen; you're just presupposing that it will.

For example, when you insert a clause into your question about the presence of the outcome by saying something like, "I'm not sure how yet" or "I don't know how this will happen," you respect your clients' struggles by acknowledging the difficulty of the miracle. You're also linguistically guiding your clients to an understanding of what's going to happen in the next part of the session, which is not a discussion about *how* to accomplish goals but a description about what difference will happen once the couple is living the reality that they desire.

Couples Therapy Isn't about Saving the Relationship

A solution focused therapist needs to be humble, and part of being humble means not overstepping the bounds of your job. It's not your role to save a relationship. If one partner says she wants to leave the relationship and you have a mindset of trying to save it, that will set you down a path of trying to prove her wrong and make her change her mind.

Instead, have the mindset that the couples' relationship is none of your business. The truth is that you don't know if staying in the relationship is a good or bad thing. Your job is to ask both partners questions about the outcome they'd experience if each of them got what they wanted.

If one client says she wants pure joy but she can only have that when her partner is out of her life, you have to trust that she can sort that out. Resist the impulse to have a conversation about *how* to make that happen. Remember, it's not your job to problem-solve, fix people, diagnose, assess, or explain to your clients what's right or wrong for them.

After the therapy, the majority of the time, couples *will* sort out their issues in a way that reconciles the relationship. But sometimes it's actually a better idea that they're not together, and that's okay. You just have to stay out of the way and trust in your clients' capability.

Protecting Autonomy in Sessions with More Than One Client

We discussed in describing the diamond stance (Chapter 5) that it's your job as a therapist to safeguard your clients' autonomy, which especially comes into play when you're working with more than one client in a session, such as in couples or family therapy. Remember that guarding a client's autonomy is one of the most important aspects within SFBT. But how do you intervene in a solution focused manner when one client violates another client's autonomy?

First of all, these violations tend to occur less frequently over the course of a session because a lot of the finger-pointing, accusations, and other frustrations among your clients are often ironed out by the end of the desired-outcome section of the diamond.

If you've done your job well, you've woven their desired outcomes together in a way that no longer makes each best-hopes answer mutually exclusive. When you can then have a conversation with your clients about what they want—a best-hopes answer that they can both buy into—you'll find that they'll most likely remain engaged and focused for the remainder of the session without saying mean and hurtful things to one another.

However, you may encounter the occasional instance when you still need to intervene. So how do you do that while remaining true to the tenets of solution focused brief therapy? You do what you've been doing all along—you take each person's answer as legitimate while also moving the conversation forward with new questions about the presence of the desired outcome.

For example, if you're working with a couple, and Partner A says Partner B is horrible because Partner B never picks up their laundry and always leaves the toilet seat up, honor Partner A's answer as the "right answer"—remember, your clients' answers are always right—then ask something that helps to move the conversation back in the direction of the desired outcome.

You could ask, "So if your partner wasn't doing those things, what would you like to see them doing instead?" Notice the key word: *instead*. That one word helps legitimize the frustrations that Partner A has been experiencing. You don't need to spend time discussing whether the accusation is true or not. It's enough that it is true to Partner A.

The word *instead* also shifts the conversation toward the change Partner A wants rather than any more time spent on elaborating on the problem. Now they'll have to focus on the opposite of what frustrates them.

"Well, I would like them to pick up their laundry," Partner A might answer.

"What difference would it make to you if Partner B started picking up their laundry?" you ask.

"I guess I'd have more time to actually appreciate who they are."

After you ask more questions that help Partner A describe who Partner B is, you can then turn to Partner B and ask, "And if Partner A started noticing these wonderful qualities about you, what would you begin to notice about them?"

"Well, they wouldn't be nagging me and yelling at me all the time," Partner B might say.

"And if Partner A wasn't nagging or yelling, what would you like to see them doing instead?"

There's that word *instead* again. Using it helps you honor each person's story while also acknowledging that something else—something better—could simultaneously happen as well.

Once you really embrace the stance of never violating another person's autonomy, and once it fully becomes a part of you and how you operate, you may not even recognize violations of autonomy when they happen anymore. Why? You simply won't engage in them. You won't be doing anything to feed them, and therefore those violations will have no room to thrive.

Going back to the same partner relationship scenario, if Partner A says, "I'm so mad at my partner because they have turned into a big jerk," you can't let Partner A's diagnosis of Partner B become your understanding of Partner B. Instead, you have to take what Partner A said and let them know you honor it while you also create a question that honors Partner B as well.

For example, you could say to Partner A, "Gosh, it must be really hard to be married to someone that you are experiencing as a jerk. If I do a good job as a therapist and you do a good job as a client, how would you rather be describing Partner B?"

"I'd rather be describing them as the wonderful partner they used to be," Partner A might answer.

"So if we had a conversation, and I'm not sure how, but it caused your experience of being married to Partner B to return to the way it used to be, back when you described them as wonderful, would you be pleased?" Do you see how that question honors both Partner A and Partner B?

But what if you had first replied to Partner A's complaint by asking, "Well, how would you rather Partner B to be?" You would sound as though you're accepting Partner A's diagnosis that Partner B is a jerk, which would offend Partner B. Instead, you need to honor both people by saying, "Gosh, it must be hard to be experiencing Partner B that way. How would you rather be describing them?" That way Partner B understands that Partner A's words about them are their own. The words don't mean that you believe Partner B is a jerk as well.

The potential for an argument starts to escalate when one client says something mean or horrible about the other one, and the therapist panics and tries to intervene by asking a seemingly innocent question that only perpetuates the fighting or name-calling.

Resist the urge to gain more clarity about the offense by asking your client to give an example. Questions like "Can you tell me about a time when that happened?" will only feed the argument.

Instead, honor the client but remove yourself a step from the derogatory language by saying, "I hear you're experiencing the other person in this way. How would you rather be describing them?"

Can you see how that immediately de-escalates the argument? The conversation pivots from "Partner B is a jerk" to "I understand you're experiencing Partner B as a jerk" to "How would you rather be describing Partner B?" Now the session will move in a direction that can change the couple's reality for the better.

"I would rather have Partner B be the loving partner that I used to know," Partner A says.

"Can you tell me about the Partner B that you used to know?" you ask.

"Well, they used to put their clothes away and not leave the toilet seat up. They took extra care to try to impress me."

"What do you notice about them that lets you know there are some pieces of the partner you married still in there?"

"Well, they don't leave their clothes on the floor every day," Partner A answers. "There are still some days where they pick up their clothes and put the toilet seat down."

Meanwhile, Partner B is listening to all of this, thinking, *Wow, Partner A still notices the good in me.* Not only is it a huge reversal in language, but it also reiterates the fact that SFBT is a co-construction. It's a language-based approach. You can deliberately insert words that shift the conversation and construct something different.

Apply your expertise in language to use terms such as *instead* and *rather be* and *experiencing* to keep the session focused on the desired outcome, then listen in amazement as your clients use their autonomy to create new and wonderful realities for themselves.

Chapter 13

Desired Outcome

Working with Children and Adolescents

Adapting SFBT Language for Children

One of the questions we regularly receive is, "How do you work with children who aren't very verbal?" Perhaps the child is very young or has a developmental delay that affects their speech or the ability to track a conversation.

In order to engage in solution focused brief therapy, the only requirement on the clients' part is to be able to answer questions. These don't have to be complicated or intense questions, but children have to be able to track a conversation well enough that if you ask a question, they'll be able to provide an answer that enables you to ask the next question.

It doesn't matter how young the kids are, as long as they can engage in that process. If they can't, however, they may not benefit from SFBT because it's a form of talk therapy.

For the children who are verbal enough to benefit from SFBT, you're going to need to obtain a best-hopes answer from them to get your session started, just like you would with any client, but you'll need to adapt the language so they understand you. They might not comprehend what you're saying if you ask, "What are your best hopes?"

Part of your responsibility as a therapist is to customize your questions as needed for each client—in this case, children—so they are more answerable.

Some of the ways that you might adapt the best-hopes question is to consider the circumstances of each child and what's important to them.

If they were brought to your office by a parent, you might be able to ask, "If you and I did a really great job today, and when you walked out, your mom (or dad) was able to see that you were happy you came, what would they see about you that would let them know you're really happy?"

Notice how that question is applicable to the child, even though their parent might also have input on what happens during therapy.

When working with children, it's also important to change the pacing of your language as you ask questions. Speak slower and in a manner that's more explanatory.

Another way you might obtain a best-hopes answer from a child is to ask something like, "If you had a great time here, what would we have done?" Or you could ask slightly older children, "If this was helpful to you, what might we have talked about?"

Again, the aim in obtaining a best-hopes answer is to establish what the client wants from this process, so your job in working with young children is to adapt that question a bit so that they can understand it.

Accept whatever answer they give you as the right answer and take it seriously, even though you might have to work hard to ask follow-up questions in order to really understand what each child's best hopes are from the session.

A Child's Surreal Best Hopes: Magic, Unicorns, and Superheroes

A Closer Look with Adam

Often when you ask children about their best hopes, they will answer with something surreal like, "I want my own fluffy unicorn."

When therapists hear fantastical answers like this, their initial reaction is often to reply, "That's impossible. You can never have that. It isn't real."

Be very careful not to discount your clients' answers in that way. Don't disbelieve them, and don't try to change their answers.

So what do you do with fantastical answers? How do you build an entire conversation around things that aren't real?

First of all, slow down the conversation and start asking other questions to help you understand why the child wants what they do. Ask about the difference it would make: "If you were able to get your very own fluffy unicorn, why would that be a good thing for you?"

Other children might answer your best-hopes question by saying they want to be superheroes. You'll also need to ask follow-up questions to find out why that's important to them. Sometimes this requires that you enter into that fantasy world with them. Again, the burden to adapt the SFBT process is yours and not theirs.

You might ask something like, "If you were Superman, what would your favorite superhero power be? Would it be X-ray vision? Would it be to be able to fly? Would it be super strength?"

Those kinds of questions will help you understand what it is about being a superhero that's meaningful to them. You'll gain clarity about what's going on in their lives and also what they're hoping to get out of life.

Maybe being a superhero means they'll get to take care of people or feel strong. Likewise, if they have a fluffy unicorn, it could mean they'll feel comforted or experience life as fun. Those are outcomes you can build a conversation around.

For example, you can transport a child who wants to have fun into lots of different arenas. You could say, "If you were able to have fun like you have with your fluffy unicorn, but you could also have that same kind of fun at school, even if your fluffy uni-corn wasn't able to go to school, what would be the first thing you would notice that would let you know this was a fun-kind-of-school day?"

Again, don't discount their fantastical answers. Work hard to understand what they're trying to convey through the language they give you. Therapists need to work very hard at not placing their own grown-up limitations on little people. Children think, act, and behave in ways that are different from us. Embrace their limitless and magical perspectives. Adapt to their creativity. We'll be amazed that kids really can be superheroes if we don't get in their way!

Acknowledging the Non-Client Parent in the Room

Let's say you're working with a young boy whose dad is also in your office, but he's an observer rather than a participant in the therapy session. Let's also say that the boy answers the best-hopes question by saying he wants his dad to come outside and play with him. When you ask what difference it would make if the dad came outside and played with him, the boy replies, "It would make me happy."

Seems simple enough on the surface, right? All you have to do is move on to the description portion of the diamond and continue the conversation. "Oh, you'd be happy," you might say. "What would you play when you are outside with your dad?" You'd ask questions with the idea that all the dad has to do is play with his son more and everyone's lives would get better. Maybe they would. Maybe the dad has just been distracted lately, but he's home enough that he just needs to engage with his son more.

On the flip side, maybe this is not so easy for the dad. After all, you don't know everything that's going on with the family. Maybe the dad has a really hard job or works multiple jobs to provide for his wife and son. Maybe he leaves early in the morning and doesn't arrive home until super late at night, when his son is already asleep. It's not fair to ask that dad to be home more. If he *was* home more, there might be serious financial consequences.

Because you don't know the full picture, it's better to err on the side of caution and ask questions about the boy's desired outcome of wanting to be happy in this way instead: "How would you show your dad that you were happy in the moments that you *do* get to see him?"

Be mindful to ask questions that put the client in a position to be successful and not ultimately create more frustration.

Adolescents Who Are Mandated to Come to Therapy

A Closer Look with Adam

You may be wondering how to get a best-hopes answer from teens who don't want to come to therapy. Maybe their parents forced them to come, or their school or a judge mandated that they attend.

There was a time in my career when I was employed at a juvenile justice detention center, a form of jail for kids ages 12 to 18 who have gotten into trouble with the law. My job was to work with them from a mental health perspective to prepare them to get out of jail and hopefully put their lives into a particular place where they wouldn't need to come back.

As you can imagine, many of the kids who were there began their relationship with me with trepidation and suspicion. When I would begin sessions with them and ask, "What are your best hopes?" oftentimes they would reply, "I don't really have any hopes" or "I just want to get out." So what do you do in this kind of circumstance?

First of all, change your perspective that just because they were told to be here that they don't want to get anything out of this process. As an SFBT therapist, you need to assume that each client you meet with—even adolescents who say they don't want to be here—has some vested interest in sticking around. Continue to ask questions that will get you to a place where you can help them to find a question that's answerable.

That might mean asking the same question multiple times but in different ways before they give a meaningful answer. As Elliott and I have talked about in previous chapters, it's essential to take into consideration the language your clients give you.

If you ask, "What are your best hopes?" and a teen replies, "I'm not very hopeful," the teen has still given you some language that you can use. They said *not very hopeful*, which also means they are a little hopeful. You can take that answer and say, "So with the little bit of hope you *do* have, what are you hoping will be useful about this conversation?"

The teen's reply might be, "I'm not hopeful about this conversation at all." You can take that language and say, "All right. So given that you're not very hopeful about this conversation, let's say this conversation *does* become a kind of conversation that gets you thinking that you might invest a little hope in this conversation. What might you come up with at that point in order to say, 'Well, I guess I really do want this one thing to come out of this conversation'?"

The teen is very likely to answer, "I just want you to stop asking me these stupid questions." The teen will try multiple tactics to get you to stop doing your job, and it's really up to you to persist.

Using the teen's language, you could say, "If somehow we got to a place in this session where I knew that somehow I didn't have to ask you any more questions, but instead you knew exactly what was going to be helpful and useful for you from our talking, how would I know? What would the signs be from you that I don't need to ask you any more questions?"

Additionally, you have the opportunity to bring up the stakeholders for this teen, like his parents or a judge or his school. You could say, "If your parents also knew that my time for asking you questions was up and I didn't need to ask you any more questions because the questions I asked had been just right for you and this mandated therapy doesn't need to happen anymore, what would they begin to notice about you that would let them know that this had been a useful mental process?"

In my example questions, you can see how important it is to take every answer adolescents give you as an absolutely perfect answer, and to take that answer and incorporate it into your next question.

The last strategy I want to mention for obtaining a best-hopes answer from a teenager is to take one step back for a bit and take the time to really get to know them and learn what's meaningful and important to them. You can then say something to the effect of, "If you and I had a conversation about what you really wanted to talk about, what would be the best thing to talk about?" This kind of question lets the client introduce you to what's important to them (let's say they respond with "video games"), and then you can ask a follow-up question like, "If we talked about video games, why would that be a good thing?" Now the conversation is off and running.

One of the kids I worked with at the juvenile detention center was really into technology, video games, and coding. So one of the things we talked about was how he got so good at these skills. He offhandedly explained, "I guess I worked hard. I practiced."

I then had proof that he was capable of practicing and putting in hard work, so I asked him, "How did you decide how to put all of that determination and practice and hard work into video games, and how did you know that was going to be a good thing for you?"

"Well, it's fun," he answered. "I like doing it."

Now he had paired "work" and "fun," so I could then take those things he had taught me about himself and put them in a different scenario and say, "Suppose you and I do work here, and somehow this work is worth putting effort into, but it's also fun work. It doesn't feel like a burden or a task. What would be a clue that would let you know this is a kind of conversation that's fun but also worthwhile to put work and effort into?"

Do you hear how taking time to understand what makes him want to work helped enable me to do my job well? That's one of the things that you need to be able to take into consideration as you conduct therapy with people—in this case, teens—who say they don't want to be here or have this conversation.

When Adolescents Want Someone Else to Change

When working with adolescents, you may also run into situations where their best-hopes answer is wanting someone else to change. They may say something such as, "I just want my parents to leave me alone" or "I want my boyfriend/girlfriend to get back together with me."

In the first chapter on desired outcomes, we talked a little about clients who initially don't take any ownership, but as this topic is especially relevant to teenagers, it's worth elaborating upon here.

So how do you have a conversation with an adolescent about someone who isn't present in the room being the person responsible to make the change? Remember, you need to take every answer your clients give you seriously.

One way to do that is to think of their answer about someone else changing and treat it as a strategy that they're presenting to arrive at their desired outcome, and not actually their desired outcome.

When you hear teens say things like, "I want my parents to let me do whatever I want," you should listen through that and hear, "I want my parents to let me do whatever I want so that I can (fill in the blank with their to-be-determined desired outcome)."

The strategy they're presenting is just a pathway to get what they really want. As a therapist, accept that answer and use it to form your next question. "So if your parents *did* let you do whatever you want, what difference would that make to you?"

Asking a question about the difference takes their strategy and moves it one step closer toward defining a best-hopes answer in which they can take ownership.

They might reply, "I guess I'd finally have freedom." You can hear in those words that they're really saying, "If my parents let me do what I want, then I'd finally be free."

Freedom is a meaningful best hope. It's a topic that can easily fill the rest of the session, and it can help shift you to a description pathway in the diamond (for example, preferred future).

You could say, "Suppose you woke up tomorrow and you had so much freedom—maybe because your parents have taken a step back, but maybe not. Regardless, you somehow felt wonderfully free. What would be the very first sign that would let you know you had that freedom?"

Notice in that language how the teen's two answers, "parents letting me do whatever I want" and "freedom," were simultaneously connected and disconnected in the phrasing. What the parents do might be connected to freedom, but it might not be. Other paths to freedom could exist as well.

Solution focused brief therapy focuses on what's truly meaningful to your clients, and if they tell you that they want someone else to change, that's because they've thought over and over, "If that person changed, I would finally get what I want," whether or not that's true.

As a therapist, you need to jump past any goals or strategies your clients may bring into the room and instead discuss the end point of their outcome—living in the reality of what they really want—not any tactics on how to arrive there.

Clients transform when they have conversations about meaningful outcomes, and those outcomes need to be realities in which they can take ownership.

Best Hopes That
Aren't Possible for Adolescents

Another scenario you might run into with adolescents is when they say they want something unattainable or something you shouldn't help them obtain. This is another subject we've addressed in earlier chapters, but it is especially applicable to teenagers.

Teens might say, "I just want to be able to play video games all day long" or "I want to stop going to school."

Presumably, those are best hopes that you can't help them accomplish. If you did, stakeholders such as parents or their school would be very disappointed with the outcome of your therapy.

Again, take their answers seriously, but view them as a strategy and not their true desired outcome. To help arrive at their true desired outcome, you could ask, "If you did get to sleep in and not go to school anymore, what difference would that make to you?"

A question about difference prompts an internal-state answer such as, "I'd finally be able to relax" or "I'd finally be happy." Those are meaningful best hopes—conversation topics that can fill an entire session and outcomes that fall within the realm of the teenager's control to create change.

If teens answer your best-hopes question by saying things like, "I want to be a movie star" or "I want to be a professional athlete," don't let yourself think or say, "That's impossible." You have no idea if you're in a room with the next glamorous movie star or star player in the NFL.

What you can do is respond by asking a question about difference, but in terms of the path to achieving their desired outcome. You might say, "Suppose you woke up tomorrow and you were on the path to becoming a movie star. What would be different to let you know that something had shifted in your life and you had taken the first step to becoming a movie star?"

Again, don't discount your clients' dreams. Maybe they'll never become a movie star or a professional athlete, but having a conversation with them about them becoming someone amazing might create change in their lives. It could spark them to become even more amazing than they already are.

Don't let seemingly unfathomable best hopes distract you. Trust that your clients know themselves better than you do. Don't trump their knowledge with your knowledge. Trust that even teenagers, maybe especially teenagers, are capable of amazing things!

Chapter 14

Desired Outcome

Working with Families

The King of the Family

A Closer Look with Adam

I used to work in a pediatric hematology and oncology unit with children who had been diagnosed with cancer. Through integrated care, I conducted therapy with these kids and their family members.

One of the families I worked with was, on the surface, a very challenging family. They consisted of a single mom who lived with four children and her own mom. Three of the children were teenagers and one was a six-year-old boy. I predominantly worked with the mom and the third child, a daughter, as well as the boy, who was diagnosed with leukemia.

When I met with this family for the first time, the boy was getting chemotherapy. I walked into the treatment room, introduced myself, and asked the family, "I'm just wondering if you can tell me what your best hopes are from our working together today?"

The little boy spoke up first and declared, "I am the king of this family."

Now this wasn't in the realm of any answer I'd been expecting. It wasn't even a goal, let alone a desired outcome. But I took him seriously and asked, "How do you know you're the king of this family?"

He lifted his chin. "I tell people what to do, and they do it."

Remember, this boy was only six years old, and he had three older siblings—all teenagers—and a mom and grandma. So I was taken a little off guard by the fact that he thought of himself as the king of the family.

"What are the king's very best hopes for our work together?" I asked.

"I want to tell you what to do, and you do it," he said.

"If I listen to what you say and do the things you say, what difference would that make to you?"

"I'd get to stay the king," he replied, as if the answer was obvious.

"And why do you want to stay the king?"

"Because it makes me happy when people do what I say."

"So if you and I have a conversation about you being happy," I asked, "would that be a good thing?"

He settled back into his chemotherapy chair. "Yeah, I want to stay happy."

I turned to his mom. "And what are your best hopes from our work together today?"

She glanced at her son, her brows knitting together. "I want to have a very good boy, someone who is kind and respectful."

"What difference would it make to you to have a boy who is kind and respectful?" I asked.

"Oh, it would make me so happy, and it would relieve so much stress. I didn't expect for my son to get cancer. I'm worried about him, and I'm concerned that this experience will teach him that he can get whatever he wants."

I understood what she was saying. In many respects, life couldn't have been easy for this young boy because of his cancer, but he was also receiving a lot of attention from it, and he seemed to be using that to his advantage.

"If you had a son who got to feel like he was a king," I asked, "maybe not the king of the family, but still a king—a kind and respectful king—would that be an okay thing for you?"

"Yes." She smiled. "I would like to live with that kind of king."

I turned to the last family member present, the teenage daughter. "And what are your best hopes from our working together today?"

She fidgeted with her bracelets. "I don't want to be overlooked," she said. "I don't want to be forgotten."

"If through this experience we made sure you weren't forgotten, what impact would that have on you?" I asked.

She glanced at her mom and brother. "I'd feel like our family was unified. There wouldn't be one person who was more important than the others, and I could care about my little brother and what he's going through without feeling resentful."

"What difference would it make to you to have a unified family where you weren't feeling resentful?" I asked.

"I wouldn't feel guilty."

"What would you like to feel instead of guilt?"

"I'd just like to be happy."

"So if we had a conversation about a reality where you got to live with a king who is kind and respectful, where you didn't get lost, and where you felt like you were part of something great, would that be good for you?"

She nodded. "Yeah, that would be good."

"And would it ensure that you didn't have to feel guilty anymore, but that you could feel connected to your family?" I asked.

"I think it would," she said.

Notice how I didn't argue with anyone in the family. Imagine how detrimental it would have been if I had argued. Imagine if I'd said to a six-year-old boy with cancer, "You don't get to be the king. Your mom is supposed to be the queen of this family."

Likewise, imagine if I'd said to the teenage daughter, "Of course you're going to feel resentful. Your little brother has cancer! Everyone's going to wait on him hand and foot, and you need to just accept that."

Instead of arguing, I held on to each family member's answers and gradually integrated them into one narrative. I took the boy's answer and built it into the mom's answer, then I built both those answers into the daughter's answer. Your job as an SFBT therapist is to weave a desired outcome from everyone present in the session. Use it to co-construct a new reality with them, like I did with this family, a reality where none of them are forgotten, where they can live with a kind and respectful king—a king who is unified with his family.

After having conversations with the king and his family over the course of one year, we were nearing the end of therapy. We had many SFBT conversations about the differences that being unified made, how the king was being kind and respectful, and how the family was supporting each other during a time of great difficulty.

When we terminated therapy, the boy was in remission from cancer and said to me during our final session, "Thank you for helping me be a good king!"

There is nothing better than interacting with a family that is capable of greatness, and in this case, a family with a good king!

Best Hopes with More Than One Person

Similar to couples therapy, in family therapy you'll be working with more than one person in a session. This could be a parent and a child, both parents and their child, just siblings, or a parent (or parents) with multiple children. This might even be a multigenerational family. Start the session at the top point of the diamond and establish a best-hopes answer for everyone present.

If you're given a strategy or goal as an answer, dig deeper to get an actual desired outcome. Also be sure that the answers aren't mutually exclusive—one person's answer shouldn't discount anyone else's.

If the answers *do* compete rather than being compatible, keep working through those answers until you arrive at combinable best hopes from each person—outcomes that are complementary.

Again, asking about difference is the key here. Difference questions spur compatible internal-state answers like peace, happiness, and satisfaction.

Weave those answers together and ask, "If we had a conversation today that led to having more peace, happiness, and satisfaction as a family—whether or not the problems you mentioned still exist—would you all be pleased?"

Let's say you're working with a parent and a child, and the parent says, "I want my child to listen and obey," but the child says, "I want my parent to get off my back."

You can reply to the parent by asking, "If your child was listening and obeying, what difference would that make to you?"

The parent might answer, "Oh, that would be such a relief. I'd be able to stop worrying. I'd finally feel a sense of unity in our family."

You can then ask the child, "And if you were able to get your parent off your back, what would be different for you?"

The child might answer, "I'd be able to do what I want to do. I'd be happy."

Note that among those answers between the parent and child, they gave the best hopes of relief, unity, and happiness—which are all compatible.

Respect is another best-hopes answer that both the parents and children often give in family therapy. The parent wants the child's respect, and the child wants the parent's respect.

After asking questions about difference—several times in some cases—you'll eventually arrive at a place of agreement.

It's not your clients' responsibility to come to therapy with a prepackaged and unified answer to your best-hopes question. On the surface, they may not all want the same thing, but it's your job to ask questions about difference that will help them articulate desired outcomes that can be woven together.

Once you do that, you can have a conversation that everyone present can invest in and agree upon—a conversation that can bring about lasting change.

When Parents and Children Are Living in Two Different Cultures

Many therapists work with families that have immigrated to the United States (or whatever country you're practicing in). As a result, you'll often meet with bicultural families. In these situations, the generation coming from the former country brings a framework for what's acceptable in a family, while the acculturated younger generation often has different expectations for what a family should be like.

For example, here in the United States, individuality and autonomy are strongly promoted and valued by young people, whereas in many other parts of the world, a sense of community takes precedence over individuality and autonomy. Consequently, among bicultural families there is a cultural component of "My child should behave in this way" versus "I don't buy into that value of my parents any longer."

These clashes can also present themselves in blended families with partners from different cultures. Each person brings their own family histories and hopes to establish them in a unified family experience, but sometimes that proves to be very difficult.

As a therapist, how do you establish compatible best-hopes answers with clients who have very different backgrounds? Honor both cultures and backgrounds. Don't take sides. Through your questions, help each client who is present understand that, as they respect and value all perspectives in the family, they can arrive in a place of unity.

A dad might say, "I want my son to be a part of my culture," while his son answers, "I want my dad to understand that I'm part of a different culture."

As you listen through each answer, hear how both the father and son want to be respected and valued and have their opinion heard.

You might ask the dad, "If you got to live according to your culture, and you could also value your son's opinions and choices, what difference would that make?"

The dad might reply, "We'd finally feel at peace with one another."

Ask the son a similar question to help him also define his own meaningful desired outcome, and weave each best-hopes answer into one narrative. Doing so will help the father and son consider the differences they would notice if each of them felt at peace and loved and respected.

When working with clients from divergent backgrounds, you'll need to get to a place in the conversation where you can ask, using the language they've given you, "If you got to live the way you want to live, how would you show him you were appreciative of being able to live this way?" or "How could you show that you were appreciative of being loved and respected and valued? Would that make a difference to you?"

In essence, you want to help each person describe the reality of living in peace as a family, a reality where each person lives according to their respective values while also acknowledging that the other family members are doing the same for themselves. This woven narrative will be the family's foundation for creating change that they all can agree upon.

Chapter 15

Resource Talk

A Diamond Description Pathway

Now that you know how to get a best-hopes answer, it's time to move on to building a detailed description of the presence of the best hope. Remember, there are three types of description: 1) resource talk, 2) history of the outcome, and 3) preferred future. The next three chapters will cover each of these description pathways. We'll start with resource talk.

The Number One
Drug Dealer in Waco, Texas

Diving Deep with Elliott

My first job in this field was at a halfway house for teens who had been incarcerated in juvenile corrections facilities in Texas—basically prison for youth. This halfway house was a transitional living facility for teens who had turned 18 and were released from prison because they had aged out of the system. The then-named Texas Youth Commission (now know as the Texas Juvenile Justice Department) required them to spend time at a halfway house before they were sent home.

The halfway house I worked at was a collection of apartments in a terrible location, right across the street from the biggest drug houses in Dallas, which couldn't have been easy for one of the kids I worked with named Little Waco.

I met him at a time in my career when I was becoming significantly better at solution focused brief therapy. I'd made strides largely because I learned how to be impressed by my clients, even people like Little Waco.

Little Waco was tall and Black and had *Waco* carved into the side of his hair. He was 18, but he had gone to prison at the age of 14 for being the biggest drug dealer in Waco, Texas. That fact was obviously concerning, but on the other hand, it was pretty impressive, and because I focused on being impressed by him, it changed the way I asked him questions.

One day during a group therapy session at the halfway house, I said to Little Waco, "Obviously dealing drugs wasn't good—look at all the trouble it caused you—but I am curious, how did you become the biggest drug dealer in Waco, Texas?"

"Can I get up and show you?" he asked. With my permission, he walked up to a whiteboard at the front of the room. "Rule one," he said as he wrote it down, "never get high off your own supply."

Now I've been a lot of things in my life, but thankfully I've never been a successful drug dealer or user, so I asked, "Why not?"

"Well, there are two reasons," he explained. "If you use drugs that you buy wholesale, then you'll be cutting into your own profit." Keep in mind this is an 18-year-old kid saying this, a kid who established these rules when he was 14. "Also, drugs alter your way of thinking, and you have to be really sharp when you're running a big enterprise because you'll be a target."

I nodded to show that I was following.

"Rule two," Little Waco said, writing it on the board with his dry-erase marker. "Diversify."

"What do you mean?" I asked.

"Don't just sell one drug. You've got to sell multiple drugs." He explained that the drug he first introduced to his gang was meth, but he later expanded with marijuana and various pills.

"Rule three," he continued, "build a staff."

"Build a staff?" I repeated, implying that I needed clarification.

"Yes. If you're going to sell drugs, you've got to take over street corners. I'm only one person, so I can only be on one street corner. But if I have lots of people working for me, we can strategically spread out to other street corners. Another benefit of having a staff is that they'll get caught with the drugs instead of you. If they do get caught, you have to immediately call them and say, 'If you don't snitch, I'll save a bunch of money to give you for when you get out of jail or prison.'" Unfortunately for Little Waco, this was the reason he was sent to prison—one of his staff snitched.

He had a few more rules and wrote them all down for the group in the room. I looked at this list and this kid, and I was honestly amazed. Someone with a seventh-grade education was telling me how to buy something wholesale and how to profit first.

Yes, Little Waco had made bad decisions, but he was also incredible, and I was concerned for him. He knew drug dealing this well, and in a couple of weeks the halfway house would be sending him home, where he would likely go back to selling drugs.

How could I help Little Waco? Well, it just so happened that he was full of resources.

I walked up to the whiteboard and erased, "Rules of Dealing Drugs," which he had written at the top of his list. I turned to him and asked, "What if I challenge you and said that I want you to sell something that doesn't have the potential to send you to prison? What would you call this list instead, and how would you change it?"

"Hmm," he said, mulling over my questions as he looked back and forth from me to the board. "I think it's the same list."

"Give me an example," I said.

He uncapped his marker and wrote at the top of the list, "Rules of Selling CDs." This was in the early 2000s, when CDs were really popular at the time.

"Can you tell me how this list is the same?" I asked.

"Well, I still can't use my own supply."

"Why not?"

"Because if I buy CDs wholesale, and I open the shrink wrap to play them, then I can't sell them anymore, so I'd be cutting into my profit."

I nodded. "What else?"

"I'd still have to build a lot of staff."

"How come?"

"I'd want my CDs in multiple malls in order to sell a lot of them, so I'd need a bunch of employees." He went on to describe in detail how he could sell CDs with the same list of rules that he'd used to sell drugs.

A couple of weeks later, Little Waco approached me in the halfway house and gave me a big hug. "Hey, Mr. Elliott," he said. "I'm being released and going back to Waco. And I hope I never see you again." I smiled because that was a good hope. No one wants to return to a halfway house.

Several years later, I found myself at a car dealership getting my oil changed. I knew I was going to have to wait for a while, and I don't sit still very well, so I went for a walk around the dealership. When I was in the used car part of the lot, a tall Black man started walking toward me.

Panic zinged through my body. I realized I was blood in the water for any salesperson, and I didn't intend to buy a car today.

The man came within 10 feet of me and paused. "Mr. Elliott?"

I shifted on my feet, disoriented. The only people who ever called me Mr. Elliott were the kids I'd worked with at the halfway house many years ago. "Yes?"

"It's me, Little Waco."

I blinked twice. He no longer had *Waco* carved into the side of his hair, and he was wearing a tie and a crisply ironed shirt, but I finally recognized him as the boy I knew when he was 18.

He started crying and rushed over, throwing his arms around me.

"Hey, man," I said, patting him on the back. "How are you doing?"

He pulled away and brushed the tears from his eyes. "I've been wanting to find you for years. After I got home from the halfway house, I realized I didn't have to sell drugs anymore. I realized I'm not good at drug selling; I'm good at selling. So when I saw a job listing for a car salesperson, I thought, *I can do that*. I'm now the head of sales here for the used car department."

Now that would have been impressive at any car dealership, but it was especially impressive at this huge car dealership.

"I have to thank you for this job," he said, weeping and hugging me again. "But that's not the biggest thing I want to thank you for."

"Oh?" I asked, curious.

"I'm married now, and I have two children. My wife doesn't know the old Little Waco. She doesn't fear that I'm going to go out and do something that could potentially get me arrested. She doesn't know the type of person I used to be. She only knows who I am today. She knows I'm a law-abiding citizen, and she never worries about me getting into trouble or going away to prison for years, and I have to thank you for that because you showed me that I wasn't a good drug dealer; I was good at sales."

Once Little Waco understood that he was good at sales, his vision expanded, and he saw other possibilities, which meant he could picture himself making a living that didn't risk sending him back to prison.

SFBT therapists often mistake resource talk for assessing clients for the resources they have. But that's not resource talk. Resource talk is about listening very closely to the evidence of the resources your clients have that can make their desired outcome—their transformation—possible.

I knew just by his circumstances that Little Waco's desired outcome was to get out of the halfway house and not come back, so through our resource talk, I had to listen really closely to the resources he had to make that possible.

One of the resources I heard from him was that he was the number one drug dealer in Waco at the age of 14. Now on the one hand, I didn't want to congratulate him for that; but on the other hand, it was important that I asked him how he did that.

I knew he must have had resources within him that, if used well, could change his life for the better. Think of Lex Luthor in the Superman comics and movies. Lex Luthor was a super brain who used his intelligence for bad things. But what if he'd had a therapist who had flipped that for him by saying, "Hey, man, you have some amazing gifts!"

Little Waco had amazing gifts too. Imagine the leadership skills he needed to do what he was doing at 14 years old. My job was to ask him questions that evoked those resources and helped him see himself differently.

If you hope to make a difference in your clients' lives, you have to make a difference with what they see in the mirror. The best way you can help people is to help them see themselves in a different and more positive way.

When Little Waco first came to the halfway house and attended group therapy, he saw a drug dealer when he looked in the mirror, but by the time he left, he saw someone who was good at sales.

That's our job as SFBT therapists—and that's the point of resource talk.

The Importance of Resource Talk

Aside from establishing a desired outcome, resource talk is the single most important part of the diamond. Learning to talk to people in a way that highlights their resources is an essential skill to master in solution focused brief therapy. People don't often think about their resources, and as they learn to identify them, they'll realize their own capacity for greatness, which they need in order to achieve change.

You might be thinking, *What about those people who have no resources?* Those people do not exist. Every human being has flaws and resources. Like we mentioned in the stance chapters, there's no perfect person on the planet. And because that's true, there's also no perfectly imperfect person on the planet.

The fact that the clients who walk into your office have lived as long as they have, no matter their age, is evidence that they have resources.

Train your brain to listen to your client's story differently. People don't think of themselves as resourceful. They carry more doubts than confidence. Resource talk provides an opportunity for them to present evidence of their greatness, and it allows you to bring their brilliance into the rest of the session. That brilliance— those resources—shows up in multiple ways.

Elliott could have decided that because Little Waco was a huge drug dealer at the age of 14, he was doomed. Instead, he decided to feel impressed and curious about how he accomplished such a feat. Little Waco was a bit like Lex Luthor, and Elliott helped him become like Superman.

The best part about resource talk is that when you talk to people about what makes them great, they transform. Likewise, the loved ones in their lives are impacted too, even if they're not in the session. Because Little Waco transformed, he made a new life for himself—one that was stable and included a wife and children. One that didn't involve persuading others to buy or sell drugs. Resource talk was the impetus for all that remarkable change.

Resource Talk: A Description of the Desired Outcome

As a therapist, you can have all kinds of resource-oriented conversations that are not connected to the desired outcome, but if you do, the conversation will turn into rapport building or "fostering a therapeutic alliance"—tactics used in other therapeutic modalities to build a relationship of trust.

Therapists like to ask their clients, "So tell me about you." And when their clients answer, therapists will pay compliments and try to relate. "Wow, that's so amazing!" they'll say. "I have a sister who also works for the government. Let me tell you about her."

But the purpose of discussing resources in solution focused brief therapy is different from other therapeutic modalities. In SFBT, you don't use resource conversations to foster a relationship with your clients; instead, you use resources to help them take responsibility—or blame—for the possibility of their desired out-come becoming a reality. Above all, remember that resource talk is a description of the desired outcome.

Asking your clients, "How did you get so good at that?" might make you sound really interested in them, which might help them feel good about you, but that's not the purpose of resource talk. The purpose is for clients to describe what they do that's consis-tent with their desired outcome. The purpose is for you to get to know that version of them, and for them to also identify that ver-sion of themselves—the version that is capable of transformation.

So how do you keep the desired outcome present during a "getting to know you" conversation? One way is to bring up the outcome straightaway by structuring your resource-talk questions around it.

For example, if your client's desired outcome is peace, you could ask, "When in your life have you felt the most peace? What did you do to ensure that this peace was present?"

However, you don't need to immediately bring up the desired outcome. Sometimes in resource talk you just gather information (resources) about the client that you'll use later on in the session.

Regardless of whether you overtly talk about the desired out-come during resource talk, your client should already assume its presence. For example, if you went to see a doctor because you hurt your knee and the doctor asked, "What did you have for break-fast?" you'd assume she's asking that seemingly random question because it must have something to do with your hurt knee.

Likewise, because you start each session by establishing a desired outcome—such as peace—then in resource talk when you ask your client, "Are you married?" there's an assumption that that question is somehow connected to your client's objective of achieving more peace.

Following is a typical transition from the desired-outcome sec-tion of the diamond to the resource-talk description pathway that naturally sets up this assumption.

You: If we had a conversation that was about the outcome you established, would you be pleased?

Client: Yes.

You: Great. Can I spend a little bit of time getting to know you?

Because the initial "getting to know you" question follows the question about having a conversation about the desired outcome, the client realizes that the resources they will then discuss will be related to the desired outcome, even without that overtly being stated by you.

What Counts as a Resource?

A Closer Look with Adam

In resource talk, you ask your clients for traits, skills, strengths, or qualities that make them great. Sometimes that means asking about important people in their life and what those people would say if you could ask them about your clients.

No matter how you phrase your questions, your aim in resource talk should be to ask your clients to share at least one positive thing that's happened in their lives, to accept blame (responsibility) for that positive thing, and to explain what it is about them that helped them manifest that positive thing.

The answer could be an outside factor like, "I have a great friend who helps me achieve things professionally," but that gives the credit to someone else, so your next question needs to bring the accomplishment back to the client: "So what about *you* makes your friend so devoted to working with you?" Your client's thinking will have to shift internally. They might answer, "I guess I'm a good friend."

At the end of a resource-talk conversation, your clients should have a mental list—in some cases a written list—of all the things that make them awesome.

Consider the following resource-talk conversation Elliott had with one of his clients.

Elliott: What's been better since we last met?

Client: I don't feel depressed anymore.

Elliott: What's made the difference?

Client: Well, I'm on medication now.

Elliott: What have you done to ensure that your medication is going to work as effectively as possible?

Client: I take it every day at the same time.

Elliott: What does it take for you to remember to take your medication every single day at the same time?

Did you notice how Elliott took the client's answer and turned it into a resource? Yes, the medication was probably helping the client, but Elliott also helped the client see what resources the client had within themself that made the medication effective, in this case timeliness and consistency.

How to Start a Resource-Talk Conversation

We've spent a lot of time in this book detailing how to begin a therapy session, which starts with asking clients about their best hopes (desired outcome). Because of that, you might find the flexibility and options within each description pathway, such as resource talk, a little jarring at first.

You may be reading this book because you were expecting the ABCs of how to do solution focused brief therapy. But there's an art to this. We're doing our best to explain that art, what it looks like, and how we got good at it, but at the end of the day some of what a therapist does in therapy comes down to the art of "peopling." You need to apply the instincts you've learned to be good with people in any given circumstance, and try not to get caught in the weeds of overthinking the mechanics.

One area that therapists get confused about is how to even begin a resource-talk conversation. There isn't one right way to do this, but how Elliott tends to make the transition from the desired-outcome section of the diamond to resource talk is he asks the client, "If we had a conversation that led to that outcome, would you be pleased?" After the client says, "Yes," Elliott says something like, "So if I set that (insert the desired outcome) aside for a second, can I take a minute to get to know you?"

During the resource talk that follows, Elliott will glean any important information he learns about his clients (skills, traits, people in their lives), and he'll put that important information in his pocket, so to speak.

For example, if a client says, "I have a roommate, and she and I do a lot of things together," he makes a mental note that the roommate is someone meaningful to the client. Later in the conversation, he can then bring up the roommate and ask something like, "What's your roommate's name again?"

"Sara," the client might answer.

"And if Sara saw you doing your desired outcome (use the client's language), what would she notice about you?"

Now he's using the roommate's perspective to accomplish resource talk, because he can use what Sara would answer about the client to describe the resources that he then can help the client take ownership of through further questions.

You can't do therapy unless you know foundational things about your clients. What do they do for a living? Where do they live? Are they religious? Are they married or single? Do they have children? Who are the most important people in their life?

If you don't happen upon information like that in the desired-outcome section of the diamond, you can ask about it in resource talk.

Resource talk comes across as a natural "getting to know you" process, but its purpose isn't to get to know your clients—it's for your clients to teach you how to ask them meaningful questions. And questions become meaningful when they're about things that are relevant and impactful to someone. During resource talk, think of your client as your educator, and you'll be surprised by how quickly this education will happen because people can't hide who they are. They tell on themselves.

For example, you might be working with a client who you have already learned is the mother of a teenage girl. "So what do you do for a living?" you ask.

"I'm an author," your client says.

"What kind of books do you write?"

"Books for young adults—teenagers." Your client has just told on herself, meaning she has revealed more than one thing about herself through one answer.

"How did you get to know teenage brains so well that you know how to speak to them?" you can then ask. Your client will give you answers of specific resources she has.

Later on, you can bring up those resources and ask a question that shows how they apply to other areas of your client's life. You could ask something like, "So since you're so good at knowing how to speak to teenagers, how do you use that skill in order to parent your daughter?"

Your client might pause before she answers because those two things—being an author who writes for teenagers and being a mom who is raising a teenager—aren't things she has normally connected. "Well, I guess I talk less and listen more," she might eventually reply.

You can then ask her something like, "And what tells you when you've listened to your daughter in just the right way?" or "What difference does it make to your daughter when you've heard her just right?"

As you can see, resource talk is twofold. It involves not only getting to know your clients but also presupposing that they can utilize skills from one area of their lives and apply them to another area.

People forget their own greatness. And as a result, they don't apply their greatness unilaterally.

You see this all of the time in therapy. Your clients will take for granted exceptional skills they possess and view them as ordinary just because those skills have become commonplace in their lives. Perhaps they've been exercising these skills for so many years that they no longer recognize them as noteworthy. They believe they're easy.

It's your job to remind your clients that if they are great enough to achieve what they've already done before, then they can inherently do more great things.

Asking for a List of Resources

The clients who come to your office aren't people who usually feel great about themselves or their lives at the present. During resource talk, it's your job to help them rediscover their greatness and the resources they do have.

If you say to clients who have hit rock bottom, "Tell me what's great about you," they would deeply struggle to have that conversation. One thing you can do in that situation is to ask them for a list of resources. Doing so applies some healthy pressure for them to answer.

You could say something like, "I noticed you work at a flower shop. Can you tell me twenty-five things you have inside you that allowed you to get so good at arranging flowers?"

Asking for those twenty-five things applies pressure for your clients to really concentrate and dig deep to find the good within themselves.

It doesn't matter if you ask for 5, 10, or 25 resources, but when your client finally answers with a list of however many resources you've asked for, you can then ask, "And if you use those skills to get through this difficult time, what difference would that make?" If you wished, you could fill an entire session with a conversation about how your clients maximize and apply their strengths.

Some therapists ask us if they or their clients should write down the list of resources. Honestly, it doesn't seem to matter. Regardless, the impact has been made. Clients change for the better.

As you transition into resource talk, be aware that resources are often difficult to discuss for most clients. People have an instinct to dampen their greatness, either because they're conditioned to be too humble or because they are in very low place in their lives right now. Your number one job is to change what they see when they look at themselves.

If a man comes to therapy feeling like a bad dad and walks out of therapy feeling like a bad dad, what are the chances he's going to behave like a good dad? Very slim.

You have to influence what he sees when he looks at himself, and that's going to require persistence on your part because people don't change how they view themselves terribly easily. Your clients are going to test you, and you need to keep pushing.

Therapists sometimes ask us, "What do you do with a client who's not proud of anything?" You push! In the words of the beloved basketball coach Jim Valvano, "Don't give up. Don't ever give up."

Whether or not the way you conduct resource talk includes asking for a list of resources, this description pathway is your opportunity to have an "I'm so amazed by you" conversation with your clients. It's how you help them assume the stance that you've taken about them before they even walked through your door. It's how you highlight their greatness and capability. When people catch the vision of their capabilities, they begin to live up to those capabilities.

"I'm Not a Good Mom!"

Diving Deep with Elliott

I saw a woman named Mila (name changed) a few years ago who was really struggling to believe in herself. She got caught using drugs in front of her children, so the state of Texas removed the children for their safety, as they should have. When I asked Mila, "What are your best hopes from our talking?" she replied, "I want to get my children back."

"How would you notice you were on a pathway to getting your children back, and what difference would that make for you?" I asked.

"I'd feel like a good mom," she said.

"And what twenty-five things do you have inside you that let you know you're capable of being a good mom?"

She glared at me and said, "Aren't you listening? I was using drugs around my kids! I'm not a good mom! I have to learn how to do it."

With great sensitivity, I asked, "So what would you call the type of mom who's been through all the things you've been through, and when the chips were down, instead of reaching for a drink, you reached for a phone and called a psychotherapist? What type of mom does that?"

Mila started weeping and answered, "A good mom."

During resource talk, the first thing we put on our list of Mila's qualities was a good mom.

No one should be defined by their mistakes; they should be defined by how they respond to them. Mila had made a very big mistake, but that's not how I was going to allow myself to define her. I defined her by how she responded to her mistake, and how she responded was coming to see a psychotherapist.

As Mila kept identifying new traits, skills, and strengths that she possessed, I watched her light up with more self-confidence. At one point she said, "I have a desire to not have my children go through what I went through."

"What did you go through?" I asked.

"My parents were abusive, and I was homeless as a child."

"So in spite of all the mistakes you've made as a parent," I said, "how did you always ensure that your children would never be homeless?"

Answering that was enlightening for Mila. Until then, she'd never viewed herself as someone with the strength and resources to always keep a roof over her children's heads.

During resource talk, it's important to not try to solve the client's problem with the resources they give you. Let the client draw these conclusions for themselves and have their own lightbulb moments. Those moments will be more meaningful that way and resonate longer.

Remember that SFBT is an approach about description. It's not about how I use Mila's resources to solve her problems. It's about how I use Mila's resources to help her describe more of her resources. She'll realize on her own what she is capable of as she applies them.

Resource talk allows clients to experience themselves in a new way. They stop living the script of "bad mom" or "addict" or "depressed person," and they start believing in themselves, which helps them start to live a new script. Mila started living the script of "good mom," and she ultimately did get her kids back.

Through resource talk, you give your clients the opportunity to answer questions that allow them to view themselves as positive. As a result, your clients gain self-confidence. As a therapist, if I can give my clients self-confidence, I feel like I've done my job. With self-confidence, they'll be able to do anything.

What Sets Resource Talk
Apart from Other Description Pathways?

In many ways, resource talk is a very unusual part of the diamond. When we teach about obtaining a description, we often infuse a timeline into it, which we'll discuss more when we examine the history of the outcome and the preferred future in upcoming chapters. For now it suffices to say that those description pathways can fit in one area of a client's timeline in life. But resource talk is different. It's timeless. It isn't limited to just the past, present, or future.

In resource talk, you can discuss resources that have been utilized in your clients' past, resources that are occurring in their lives right now, or resources they can use in the future, like Elliott did when he asked Little Waco, "If you're selling something different from drugs, what would be different for you? How would you use the resources you have?"

When trying to distinguish the various description pathways in the diamond, it may be helpful to think of the preferred future (the topic of Chapter 16) as a description that goes into the future, history of the outcome (the topic of Chapter 17) as a description that goes into the past, and resource talk as a description that goes into the person.

Because of the internal nature of resources, you'll find that they crop up frequently during a therapy session, even if you aren't in the resource-talk section of the diamond. Regardless, learn how to listen with an ear attuned to resources.

For example, let's say that during the desired-outcome section, you ask your client, "What are your best hopes?" She answers, "I really want my husband to be happy again." Because she has told you in her very first answer that she has a husband and she cares enough about him to want him to be happy, you can hold on to that for a moment and ask, "And if your husband was happy, what difference would that make to you?"

From there, you'll establish the desired outcome; then, if you choose, you can immediately transition into resource talk by saying something like, "You mentioned you have a husband." You can follow that with questions pertaining to the husband's perspective of the wife's resources, or questions that lead to why he matters to her.

A resource is anything that's important to your clients. The ability to achieve a feeling can even be thought of as a resource. Why? Because what your clients want (their desired outcome) is something that they have felt before—remember, you can't crave what you've never tasted—and because they've felt it before, they must have some know-how, some resource, about how to create it again. Your questions will help them describe how they did it.

If the desired outcome is peace, you can ask, "When was peace in your life previously? What did you do to make that happen?"

Some therapists get confused about how questions like that, which reference the past, are resource-talk questions rather than history-of-the-outcome questions. Let's take a moment to explain the difference between these two description pathways.

Resource-talk questions are about your clients' internal relationship with their desired outcome, whereas history-of-the-outcome questions are about your clients' external relationship with their desired outcome. A history-of-the-outcome conversation might look like this:

You: When was the last time you had peace?

Client: When I was in college.

You: If I had met you back then, when you had peace back in college, what would you tell me was happening that was evidence that peace was present?

You could additionally ask: "How did important people in your life notice you had peace?"

A resource-talk conversation might look like this:

You: When was the last time you had peace?

Client: When I was in college.

You: If I had met you back then, when you had peace back in college, what would you tell me you had inside you to let you know you were capable of peace?

Resource-talk questions don't need to be framed in the past, however. You can just as easily ask, "What are some qualities you have inside you that let you know you are capable of peace?" The important part is focusing on what's within your client.

If you were to ask a woman, "Are you married?" and she answered, "Yes, I'm married to a man named Curtis," Curtis is not the resource; your client's love for Curtis is the resource—the love that lives inside her—and it's related to the role she fulfills as his wife.

Likewise, if your client is a teacher, his students aren't the resource; his relationship with the word *teacher* is the resource. The fact that he has accepted the role of teacher guides several things he does in his life, and the resource is the fact that he can do those things.

For clients who are struggling to think of reasons why they're great, asking them about another person's perceptions of them can help unlock answers, especially if that person is important to them.

For example, you could ask the teacher client, "What do your students notice about you that lets them know you're doing wonderful things to help them?" and "How did you get so good at those things?" and "What did you do to convince them you were good at those things?"

People's brilliance leaks out and shows up everywhere in their lives. The wife and the teacher in the examples above have other roles in their lives too, and their strengths in one area can help them in all areas. Your questions can help illuminate those for them.

Finding Your Client's Currency

Diving Deep with Elliott

As a human being, you've trained all your life to pick up on cues from other people. When you walk into your home or your workplace, you instinctively get a sense of what's going on. Facial expressions and other indicators from people you know help you take in the situation. You innately understand what to emphasize and what to leave alone.

That same sense is what you're tracking during resource talk, except with people you don't know. When do they light up? When do they want to share more? When do they give you cues that they don't want to discuss a certain subject?

When they *do* light up, pay attention. Find out why they did and give them all the credit for how they can continue to make that "light up ability" come about in their lives.

When I was 15, I had a huge crush on a girl named Sadie (name changed), and we went on the most innocent group date together with our friends to see the movie *Twister*. I sat next to Sadie in the theater, and all I could think about was how much I wanted to hold her hand.

I started watching for clues that she might want to hold my hand too. She began to lean sideways toward me. She moved her tub of popcorn to the left, and I was sitting to her right. Those little indicators told me, *Sadie likes me!*

As a therapist, you also need to cue into the little indicators that signify what matters to your clients. Who are they willing to do anything for? For some, it's their pets that matter most. When you pull the right lever, people are willing to do whatever it takes to make dramatic changes in their lives.

Money can be that lever of change for some people. Adam's not one of those people, and that's not to say he doesn't enjoy money, but it's not what motivates him. Discussing it would not produce a meaningful conversation or budge him in a new direction.

Over the years, I've seen professionals say to Adam, "If you do the things I want, it will be good for your career," meaning it will make him more money. But that doesn't sway him one iota. His love for his family is his lever of change. He'll do anything for Becca, Rachel, Toby, and Julia.

Therapists ask us, "What do you do if you get to the end of a solution focused conversation, and the client says, 'Well, thanks for the chat, but what did that do for me?'" That tells us you didn't find your client's "currency," so to speak (one of the three indicators of establishing a meaningful best hopes, as mentioned in Chapter 11). Their currency is what's important to them, what drives them, and what they base their life decisions around. But if you find that currency—if you pull that lever of change—then at the end of your session, your client will feel the movement that just happened: the pebble in the pond that caused a ripple.

Resource talk can be 30 seconds, 5 minutes, or it can fill a whole session. You can take the resources the client has shared and transition them into the future through a preferred-future (Chapter 16) description: "Suppose you woke up tomorrow and all of those things that we just talked about were back in your life. What would you notice?" Conversely, you can take those resources and put them in the past through a history-of-the-outcome (Chapter 17) description: "When did you have these things most in your life?"

The bottom line is, even if you only spend 30 seconds in resource talk, you'll learn to be a better "question asker" because now you understand what motivates each unique client.

Resource Talk Can Be Simple

Be careful of asking your clients things like, "Can you tell me the most amazing thing you've ever done?" They'll most likely answer, "Nothing." Remember that you're meeting people at a point in their lives when things got hard, and that skews their perspective of themselves.

It's better to ask something like, "What thing in your life are you most proud of?" By phrasing your question with "most proud," it's harder for your client to answer, "Nothing," because even if the highest thing they ever achieved was a third-grade education, that's what they'll answer with: "Well, I got out of the third grade." The resources it took for them to do that are something you can build a conversation around.

When working with couples, Elliott likes to ask, "What thing about your partner do you appreciate the most, or love the most, or are the most proud of?"

Sometimes therapists think they have to ask grand questions in resource talk such as, "What is your proudest achievement?" but resource talk doesn't often begin that way. It usually starts simply, just like a regular conversation would, with something like, "Where are you from?"

Most "getting to know you" questions can lead to discussing resources. "Where are you from?" can easily lead to "Did you like it there? What did you like the most about living there?" And that can lead to "Well, I had some good friends there. My best friend was named Heidi."

To use another example, if you ask, "What do you do for a living?"—that can lead to "I'm a lawyer," which leads to "Are you good at it?"—which leads to "I guess I'm pretty good," which leads to "How did you get so good at it?"

Elliott conducted therapy with a man named Jack (name changed) and spent a large portion of the session doing resource talk with him. Jack was addicted to crystal meth and left his two kids when they were babies. When he finally decided to come to therapy, he wasn't even sure if he wanted to get clean but was mandated by a court to attend therapy. He was working as a male prostitute to make money to buy drugs.

Elliott didn't know any of those things before Jack walked into his office, and when he did learn them, Elliott didn't let them define Jack.

Jack mentioned that a positive change he'd like in his life would be to stop using drugs. Elliott asked, "What would you be doing instead of using drugs?"

"I'm into cars and all that sort of stuff," Jack said.

"Are you really?"

"Yep."

"What do you do with these cars? Do you work 'em?"

"Yeah, buy and sell them."

"What kinds of cars are you most interested in buying and selling?" Elliott asked.

"Cheap ones," Jack replied.

"Make money on those, I would guess?"

"That's right, yeah."

"And you work on them yourself?"

"Yep."

Elliott went on to ask Jack about what he did with the cars after he fixed them up. Jack answered that he would make more money.

"When you had this money, what would you be most pleased to do with it?" Elliott asked.

"Spend it on my daughter," Jack said. (Jack didn't currently have custody of his son, so it wasn't possible for him to spend money on him. However, the son did come up later in the session.)

After they talked about cars some more, Elliott asked, "Where did you learn to work on cars like this?"

"I learned from my dad when I was younger," Jack said.

"Are you good at it?"

"Pretty good."

"So if I asked you to work on my car, for example, and there was some sort of mysterious problem about it, would you just keep—?"

"I would find out what it is wrong without a computer, because a lot of people just plug a computer into a car and figure out what the problem is. I'm not like that. I want to know how it works and why it does what it does."

"What is it about you that makes you able to do that?"

"My sort of outlook on life is that it doesn't matter what it is or if I haven't done it before. I just say that I have, just to prove to myself and to everyone else that I can do it."

You can see how everything they talked about was simple things, like working on cars, but through talking about them, Jack revealed his resource of determination, and he introduced Elliott to his dad and his daughter, who are very important people in his life.

Jack went on to discuss how he wanted to make his daughter proud of him and how he wanted to show that he was also proud of her by "giving her things" and "spoiling her" with the money he earned from selling cars.

He also talked about how his dad died when he was younger, but he remembered him as being a positive person who genuinely supported him. "He was the person to sort of push me to everything that I should be doing right and not wrong," Jack said.

By the end of the session, Jack was describing in beautiful detail how he could use his resources to achieve the self-transformation that he really desired in life. He wanted to pass on the legacy that he gained from his dad to his daughter.

Jack admitted that he hadn't done a good job of that, because he left his daughter when she was a baby. But now that she was back in his care, he resolved to do better.

What's really meaningful to people bleeds into every area of their lives. So don't worry if resource talk starts out mundane. Soon enough you'll key into things like "Dad is important" and "Daughter is important," and before you know it, the client—in this case, Jack—will discover newfound hope and confidence. He'll be describing a reality where he shows his love for his daughter by passing on the legacy he learned from his dad.

Building Rapport in
Solution Focused Brief Therapy

Diving Deep with Elliott

You might be wondering how to build a therapeutic relationship with your clients when you only conduct a few sessions with them in solution focused brief therapy. Once you establish that you have belief and faith in your clients, the therapeutic relationship is actually built very quickly.

I experienced this for myself while I was on a trip to Philadelphia. I'd injured my finger and had to go to a hospital emergency room. Exhausted and irritated, I sat in the waiting room all through the night until a room could open up for me.

When I was finally taken back to one, a really wonderful doctor instantly connected with me, and the way she did that was by conveying, "I know you've had a rough night, and I'm going to do my very best to take good care of you." Instantly, we had a relationship.

Therapists have a misconception that it takes weeks to build rapport. It doesn't. It literally took seconds for me to feel connected with this doctor, and that was after being in the waiting room for 10 long hours, without anything to drink and being completely irritated.

So don't let yourself think that you can't build a relationship quickly. Relationships are built simply by taking the stance that you truly want to connect with your clients, that you truly like them. I didn't feel like this doctor was treating me like the next patient on her list. I felt like she was talking to me, Elliott, and that she was honored to do so.

Practice, Practice, Practice

Practice resource talk in your everyday life. Ask family or co-workers or friends how their day was. If they say, "It was good," ask what they did to make it good. Likewise, you can also bring up something they do that amazes you and ask them how they got so good at it.

Keep the conversation simple and casual. Learn how to speak with people about the positive things in their lives. Ask questions that help them see how they contributed to make that happen. Purposefully observe their greatness and have conversations that highlight it.

You'll learn by practicing resource talk how you have to adapt it to every person. It will be completely different each time. You'll find that some people are forthcoming. Some are reluctant. Some don't like to talk about themselves. Each person has a unique personality, and therefore you'll need to tailor your questions just right for them. Again, there's no A-B-C formula to doing this. Resource talk is a task, an art, a discipline.

It helps people to see the hero within themselves—someone with the strengths, qualities, characteristics, and skills necessary to achieve whatever their best hopes are in life.

Chapter 16

Preferred Future

A Diamond Description Pathway

This chapter will cover material that most people are familiar with if they know anything about solution focused brief therapy. However, please remember that we asked you at the very beginning of this book to set aside everything you know about psychotherapy, and about SFBT, while reading this book. This chapter may feel a little familiar, but you should proceed with care—you're going to hear about the preferred future (what many people think of when they hear the term *miracle question*) in a new way—as a description method for the desired outcome.

The Dope Sick Client

Diving Deep with Elliott

Early in my career, a mother called me and said her 19-year-old daughter, Mary (name changed), was addicted to heroin and heavily abusing it. She asked if I could help her get clean.

When Mary came to my office for the first time, I began our session by asking, "What are your best hopes from our talking?" She told me she was a freshman in college, and she wanted to become an attorney.

Now imagine someone with track marks all over their arms telling you that they want to become an attorney. In my head I thought, *There is zero chance that this person is going to be an attorney. I'm not even sure she will ever be clean from heroin. How on earth can she expect me to help her with what she wants?*

I admit I wasn't confident when I asked Mary, "What difference would it make for you to become an attorney?"

"I'd be happy," she answered. "It's the job I've wanted to do since I was a kid."

I so badly wanted to exclaim, *Then get clean from heroin and maybe you'll have a chance!* Instead, I simply said, "Suppose you woke up tomorrow and you were on your way to doing the job you've wanted to do since you were a kid. What would you notice?"

Mary co-constructed a preferred-future description with me about what it would look like to be on the pathway to becoming an attorney.

We scheduled a follow-up session, and when that time and day came, Mary didn't show up. I thought maybe she was lost. She'd only been to my office once before. I walked into the parking lot to see if any cars were circling the area—maybe I could wave her down—but I still couldn't find her. When I came back into the lobby of my office, I noticed someone was in the women's bathroom. The door was shut, and the bathroom light was shining under the crack of the door.

I waited in the lobby and finally Mary came out of the bathroom, now 25 minutes late for our appointment. She came into my office, and we did a follow-up session that only lasted 20 minutes because that's all the time we had left. That was the last time I saw her.

Mary called me a month later and apologized for being late to our last session. She confessed that she had been shooting up in the bathroom.

Now you might be wondering, *How do you do therapy with someone high on heroin?* Well, if you know anything about heroin, you know that people only get high the first time. They continue using so they don't get dope sick. Mary was using heroin to avoid feeling that way.

She apologized and said, "I'll call you in the future when I need another session."

I didn't hear from her again for about eight years, and then I received an invitation for her law school graduation. It included a handwritten note from her. She told me that if it hadn't been for the sessions I had done with her, she never would have believed she could become an attorney. And without that hope, she never would have been able to break her addiction.

That was the moment in my career when I realized that these descriptions in solution focused brief therapy really do lead toward change. SFBT descriptions aren't about superficial things changing for your clients; they're about what's really foundational and motivational for your clients—what's in their hearts becoming their realities.

Although I didn't have confidence in Mary's transformation at the beginning of our first session, I pushed past my doubts and went on to co-construct with her a meaningful description of her preferred future. And despite Mary's setback after our first session, hope took root in her and she changed into the person she wanted to be.

Misunderstanding the Miracle Question

As a therapist, you're probably familiar with the miracle question, but if not, here's a quick refresher. The miracle question is a type of preferred-future question that asks clients to consider the difference(s) they would notice in their lives after their desired outcome is present.

Like any other preferred-future question, the miracle question includes the following components: 1) the change happens spontaneously and all at once, 2) the change—a.k.a., "miracle"—happens at a time that is outside the awareness of your clients so that they have to discover the presence of the desired outcome, and 3) the change happens sometime in the future, most often the day after the current conversation.

Insoo Kim Berg developed the miracle question when she was conducting a session with a client while her team observed behind a one-way mirror. Insoo asked the client to think about the difference they would notice if the goal (the term used at the time) were completed. The client responded that they were unsure what would be different.

Out of persistence, Insoo got creative and asked a different version of the same question, which became what we know as the miracle question: "Suppose you went to sleep tonight and a miracle happened while you were sleeping. The miracle was that all of the problems that brought you here were solved and no longer a problem. What would be the first thing you would notice that would let you know this miracle had occurred?"

The client was finally able to answer the question.

Since Insoo's team was constantly looking to implement things that worked in therapy, they decided to ask another client this same question and had more success. The miracle question grew in popularity until it was widely used by all SFBT clinicians.

When we first learned solution focused brief therapy, we were taught that, in order to be doing it, we had to be asking the miracle question. That line of thought is what has led others to believe the misconception that SFBT is about the future. It's not. SFBT is about details and language and change.

Therapists often ask us, "What about clients who can't think about the future?" and "What about the future of the problem?" When we first heard these questions many years ago, they caused us to take a step back and reevaluate the miracle question. We realized that people were misunderstanding it.

The miracle question is just a way to ask about the preferred future; it's not the *only* way to ask about it. On the same note, the miracle question is just a way to do a description; it's not the only way to do one.

In line with Insoo's method, SFBT therapists were originally instructed to ask the miracle question by saying, "Suppose you went to sleep one night and a miracle happened that solved all your problems. When you woke up the next day, what would you notice?"

But early on for us, it was clear that if we said, "Suppose you woke up on the day that all your problems were solved," we were still inviting clients to be in verbal contact with their problems, and we didn't want them to be reminded about their problems at all.

Consequently, we changed our language to the following: "If you went to sleep one night and a miracle happened that made your desired outcome a reality, what would you notice?"

At first, that seemed better, but then we had a huge realization— if we went into every session planning to say, "Suppose you went to sleep one night and a miracle happened," we would be relying on a cookie-cutter technique, and in doing so, we wouldn't be allowing our clients to be part of the co-construction process.

This realization was an integral step that led to us developing our own branch on the solution focused tree, as opposed to the original Milwaukee style created by Insoo and Steve de Shazer.

What's critical to remember is that in order to allow your clients to co-construct the preferred future—or any description pathway, for that matter—you need to use their language to transition from the desired outcome to the preferred future.

Using the word *miracle* isn't necessary. You don't even need to ask any iteration of the miracle question (although it still remains the most common transitional question in SFBT).

When asking questions to co-construct a description of the preferred future, here are the key things to remember:

- Use the client's exact language of the desired outcome.

- Set the stage so the presence of the desired outcome appears suddenly and all at once.

- Ensure that the client is in the business of discovering that the desired outcome has appeared by asking the client questions that help create a step-by-step description of the differences that result from the desired outcome being present.

- Ensure that the client is the only person/thing that is changed by the "miracle," meaning that the problem still exists, but the client now has the ability to interact with the problem differently.

When you have these kinds of powerful preferred-future conversations with your clients, not only will they realize that pieces of their desired outcome are often already occurring, but they will also realize that they already know how to move forward toward their best hopes in a meaningful way.

Reiterating the Importance of a Meaningful Desired Outcome

In the first desired-outcome chapter, we introduced a client named Laura who has a nonverbal son with a severe brain injury. If you remember, Laura established that her desired outcome was to be a normal mom, but the first thing she answered when Elliott asked her the best-hopes question was, "I want to hear my son call me Mom."

If Elliott had accepted that initial response as her desired outcome, he might have gone on to ask her, "Suppose you woke up tomorrow and a miracle happened that caused your son to be able to call you *Mom*. What would you notice?" He would then have tried to conduct a description from that point forward.

Laura would probably answer with something like, "Well, that *would* be a miracle." Automatically, she wouldn't perceive this preferred future as real. Why? Because Elliott hadn't asked about the true outcome she wanted. In this imagined scenario, he hadn't worked enough to establish that what she really wants is to be a normal mom, whether or not her son ever calls her *Mom*.

This is why it's so important that you keep asking desired-outcome questions until you arrive at a meaningful outcome that could actually happen, because your clients are going to experience the descriptions you will co-construct with them as real or not depending on that outcome.

If Elliott had pushed forward in this session with Laura using the unrealistic outcome of "I want to hear my son call me *Mom*," he wouldn't have been able to have a conversation that would make a difference for her. He would get stuck because Laura would get stuck.

Remember the stance to trust in your clients' capability. If they're struggling to do the description, it's not because of their capability; it's because of your questions. You probably haven't established a meaningful enough desired outcome. Your clients are limited in how deeply they can participate because you haven't connected the conversation to something that they actually want and can realistically obtain.

When you ask questions that are connected to the outcome that your clients came to therapy wanting, they are going to engage in a deeper way and be much more able to come along with you for the description journey.

In other words, if you don't have an effective outcome, it's almost impossible for the client to do a transformative description, but if you do have an effective outcome, it's almost impossible for the client not to engage and transform.

So how do you recover from asking a bad question? You ask another question, or you go back to the desired-outcome portion of the diamond and simply ask, "So what are your best hopes again?" Don't be afraid to start over if you need to. There will be times when you think you have a meaningful best-hopes answer but don't. It's perfectly fine to recrystallize the desired outcome.

Preferred-Future Example with Laura

The following is an excerpt from another session Elliott conducted with Laura in which he demonstrates how to co-construct a preferred-future description. Remember that Laura's desired outcome is to feel like a normal mom. Also, to show how the word *miracle* isn't necessary, Elliott deliberately doesn't use it in his questions.

Elliott: Let's suppose you woke up tomorrow and for whatever reason, the normal mom feeling had found its way into your life, even with your son unable to utter the word *Mom*. What would you notice?

Laura: I guess just the buzz of the rest of the house would be going on.

Elliott: And what would be a clue that this buzz in the rest of the house really fit in with the normal mom feeling you were having when everything else is the same? Your son's condition hasn't changed, and your husband and other children are doing their typical routine. The only thing that's changed is that you feel like a normal mom. How would you know that this was a buzz that just fit with that normal-mom feeling that you would have that day?

Laura: Hmm, I've spent so much time *not* feeling like a normal mom that I actually have to think about this for a minute.

Notice that in order to make the miracle realistic, Elliott left everything else in Laura's life the same. The only thing that changed is the feeling within her. Remember, the miracle is not about changing the client's life; it's about changing the client's *perception of who they are* within their life—this will change the description of their world.

Also note that Laura had a hard time answering Elliott's question. In this case, he was thinking, *Good. That means I've asked her a meaningful question that's going to require her to give this some thought.*

Remember that SFBT is a change-oriented approach. If your clients have to think about their answer, they are also having to articulate something in a way that they never have before. This means that change is happening in this very moment.

It's okay if your client is stumped for a minute and they answer with a form of "I don't know." That response usually means one of two things: you've asked a really good question, something your client has not spent a lot of time thinking about before; or you've asked a really bad question.

The quickest way to test which is which is to say, "What do you think?" If your clients are willing to do more thinking, you've probably asked a question that they haven't thought about before, which you should recognize as a good thing.

Remember, if your clients are going to change the way they perceive themselves within their world and change the way they describe their world, it's going to take them a minute to find the words to do so. Don't for a nanosecond doubt their capability.

Laura wasn't having a hard time answering Elliott's question because she's incapable. She was having a hard time because he asked her a really difficult question, and she doesn't have a canned, carbon-copy, ready-to-go answer because she's never considered it. She has to dig deep to create this new reality, which is actually wonderful. In our approach, these moments are priceless.

Laura: I still don't know the answer.

Elliott: What do you think?

Laura: Everything is so not normal that to imagine normal . . . I just don't know.

Elliott: So if in all of the "not normal"—your son still has the brain injury and you still have hard things to manage with his condition throughout the day—if in that "not normal" you had that very clear feeling of "In spite of everything I'm dealing with, I feel like a normal mom," how would you notice it?

Laura: Well, if all the things around me stayed the same, I guess how I see things and how I think would be different.

Elliott: What would be your first clue that you were seeing things and thinking about things in a different way—a way that just kind of fit with you feeling like a normal mom?

Laura: I think I'd have to reevaluate what my perception of a normal mom is, because when I say, "normal mom," I think about how I am a mom to my other children, which is normal. It's the way all moms are with their children. But with my [nonverbal] son, I feel like his manager because I have to manage his care and therapy and appointments and medications. There's such a small amount of actual mom stuff among everything else I do for him. So I guess I would have to reevaluate.

Elliott: And what would be a sign to you that you were reevaluating in a way that you were pleased with?

Laura: Well, first I'd actually have to think about it because I don't do a lot of thinking. I'm just doing a lot of doing. But now that you've asked, I guess I'd stop and think about it.

Elliott: And how would you know you were thinking about this in particular—in a way that was changing the way you perceive "normal mom"?

Laura: I guess what makes me a normal mom for my other kids is meeting their needs. My [nonverbal] son's needs are different, so they get met differently, but the fact that I'm still meeting them is what a normal mom does. Even if some things I have to do are not normal, that doesn't mean that I'm not being a normal mom.

Elliott: Yeah, so what I think I hear you saying is, "I can do abnormal things but still be meeting the need, which is a very normal thing." Is that right?

Laura: Yeah. I guess it's a normal mom thing to take care of a child, even if the care requirement is different.

Elliott: And how would you notice that you were starting to realize on this particular day that you're doing abnormal things to accomplish a very normal task?

Laura: Well, I would notice on this day—if this day was really different—while I was doing the abnormal tasks, I wouldn't be wrapped up in feeling so angry that I have to be doing them.

Elliott: What would you be thinking about instead of the anger? What would you be thinking about when you realize, *Oh, I'm just doing abnormal mom things to accomplish very normal mom tasks?*

Laura: Maybe I'd be more engaged in what my other kids are doing. Maybe just talking about their homework or whatever they've got going on. Maybe I'd just be a little more engaged in conversation rather than getting lost in my own head.

Elliott: Would you be pleased about that?

Laura: Oh, yeah. Being angry is hard, tiring work.

Elliott: And who in your home would be the first person to notice that something had changed in the way that you felt about your "mom-ing"?

Laura: Maybe the oldest of my three kids.

Did you notice how Elliott kept asking questions about Laura's desired outcome—how she would experience being a normal mom? He wasn't trying to get her to do anything. He resisted the urge to point out, "Don't you see how you're doing normal mom things already?" If he *had* pointed that out, she would have had the opportunity to reject it. And if she's like most human beings, she would have.

Did you catch the beautiful moment when Laura had the realization for herself that she was being a normal mom because she was taking care of her kids, even if that care looked different with how she mothered her nonverbal son?

When your clients come to realizations like this on their own, they remember them. They impact them and foster change. Your clients are the architects and the experts of their own lives. Respect that by giving them the autonomy necessary to make their own discoveries in the session.

Making the Miracle
Independent of External Factors

Diving Deep with Elliott

We've discussed several times the importance of establishing a realistic and meaningful desired outcome. In the same vein, it's equally important to co-construct the miracle in the client's preferred future in a way that's independent of external factors.

Let's say I'm working with a client named Seth. If I asked him, "What are your best hopes from our talking?" and he answered, "I want to win the lottery," I wouldn't say, "Suppose you woke up tomorrow and you won the lottery . . ." Instead, I'd ask, "What would you purchase with the money?"

"I'd buy my mom a new house," Seth might reply.

"What would it be like for you to buy your mom a new house?" I'd ask.

"Oh, it'd be a glorious feeling."

"And how would your mom respond to that?"

"She'd probably cry."

"What would that do to you?"

"I would just feel so proud."

"So suppose you woke up tomorrow, feeling that glorious feeling and that pride, even before you won the lottery . . ."

That's how you go about co-constructing a preferred-future description. It shouldn't be dependent upon something else happening in your client's life. The miracle should be an entity in and of itself.

The miracle can happen whether or not the client wins the lottery. It can happen whether or not Laura's son says *Mom*. It can happen whether parents are kinder or spouses are more affectionate or bosses are more supportive.

What really drilled this idea home for me is when I was in London watching Chris Iveson conduct therapy. When he asked the client the miracle question, "Suppose a miracle happened and you woke up the next day, what would you notice?" the client understood it as a miracle that happened to the world, not just to him. When Chris further asked him what he'd notice on his way to work, the client answered, "My favorite parking spot would be available."

"No, this is something that just happened to you," Chris clarified. "Everything else stays the same. So let's imagine that on this particular day, the only parking spot available is the one farthest away from your office door, and the weather is so bad that it's pouring rain. What would you notice then that would let you know that you were still at your very best in spite of everything else around you going wrong?"

That's when I realized: Wait a minute, the miracle isn't about everything in the client's life being good. Instead, the miracle is about the client being who they want to be no matter what else is happening around them. The miracle is completely unconnected to the world and what the client wishes those external factors could be like.

So as you phrase your questions, keep the client's world normal. The only change is that the desired outcome is suddenly present, and that desired outcome is something internal for the client, something they can actualize, something that can happen tomorrow—even if that change simply means being on the path toward achieving it.

The Immediacy of the Preferred Future

A Closer Look with Adam

As Elliott mentioned above, when we co-construct a preferred-future description, it should be one that's suddenly present for your client, often something that can happen tomorrow. That level of immediacy is part of the miracle.

Immediacy is valuable because it introduces the change your clients are looking for straightaway. This means immediately they can start noticing signs that the life they are hoping for is present. Immediately they can start acting on that change. Immediately they can start behaving consistently with the version of themselves they would like to be.

Like all description pathways, the preferred future is a co-constructed conversation about difference. Additionally, the preferred future consists of language that creates a new reality. Because of those things, you need to be extra vigilant to be sure to introduce language that is consistent with your clients' desired outcome.

When your clients walk out of your office at the end of the session, they will be different, and you want that difference to be in line with the difference they are aiming for.

Sometimes during a session your clients' language will shift. They will move from talking about the desired outcome with future-tense language and suddenly shift to present-tense language.

They begin answering questions like, "Who would be the first person to notice this difference?" with answers like, "Well, my husband always notices when I do that. He loves to see me happy and tells me how happy he is when I'm happy." Notice that the future-tense question was answered with present-tense language.

When the miracle is discussed in immediate, present-tense language, your clients can begin describing the difference and, in turn, become different in the way they want to be right there in your office. They then get to take this difference with them when they leave your office.

While immediacy is important, the client's preferred future doesn't always have to be immediately possible. Think of Elliott's sessions with Mary, who was addicted to heroin. She wanted to become an attorney, but she was only a freshman in college. She couldn't have actually become an attorney by the next morning. That's why Elliott asked her questions about a preferred future that could begin tomorrow but was also a future about her being on *her way* to becoming an attorney and the difference that would make in her life.

Remember, what's really essential in a preferred-future description is the *change* related to the desired outcome being present. This means you can say something like, "Suppose you woke up tomorrow and a change has happened, the change being that now your life is different and you are on the path to (insert the desired outcome). What is the very first thing that would let you know that you are on the path toward (insert the desired outcome)?"

Notice in the phrasing that the change is something that happened all at once—the immediacy of the change is noticeable right when the client wakes up—but the difference is that life is now in line with the desired outcome. However, the *full* desired outcome isn't necessarily present.

There are times that you can jump forward beyond tomorrow when co-constructing a preferred-future description with your clients, but those situations are rare. It's much more important to keep immediacy in mind as you conduct SFBT. Clients don't want to change in days, months, or years down the road. They want to change *now*, and your job is to ask questions that help them articulate how that change can begin tomorrow. A key point is that clients don't have to wait for something else to happen or change first (e.g., "When X happens, I will finally be happy"); change can happen in an instant, and it might just be *this* instant.

The Session Itself Is the Intervention

Diving Deep with Elliott

One of the things I love most about working with Adam is that he's a therapy linguistic super nerd. He and I taught together for the first time in Bakersfield, California, several years ago, and I remember him telling the audience, "In Elliott's work, the session is the intervention." It was the first time he had said that, and it highlighted something that we both had been doing in our work, though I didn't realize it until he articulated it in that moment.

Sometimes therapists conduct a therapy session for the purpose of assigning an intervention or homework assignment. The therapist listens to the content well enough to understand how to prescribe something for the client to do after they leave the session. However, we believe that the session itself is the intervention. Because SFBT happens through language, as the client describes change and difference in great detail, change (or intervention) is happening. We don't need to wait to prescribe change, because the client's reality is changing, their perception of the problem is changing, and their vision about the way forward is changing, all because they are describing change in great detail. The more detailed a session you can have with a client, the more likely that client is to experience change, because describing the presence of the desired outcome is literally how clients change in solution focused brief therapy. Details are profound for the human brain.

I really love to cook, and I remember one time my buddy called and said, "Hey, I want to make dinner for this girl I'm dating, and I like your lasagna. Can you please share the recipe?"

"Sure," I said, and I gave it to him.

He went to the store, got all the ingredients, and called me back again when he was making it. He asked question after question so he could cook it just right. One and a half hours later, by the time I got off the phone after coaching my friend, I was really craving lasagna. Why? My brain had gone through every step and detail of preparing it.

That's what detailed descriptions accomplish for our clients. If you talk to them about the version of themselves that is sober, it makes them crave sobriety.

I've already told you the story of Mary, the freshman in college who was addicted to heroin. I worked with another woman who also was addicted to heroin, and in our therapy session we co-constructed a description of the day she was going to wake up sober. We spent about 40 minutes describing that day in extraordinary detail.

She scheduled another session for two weeks later, and when the time came, she didn't show up. I tried to call her, but her phone was out of service.

A month later, she called and said, "Sorry I missed the session. I was in rehab. I'm out now, and I've been clean for twenty-eight days."

"What happened to help you get clean?" I asked, impressed.

"I just kept thinking of myself as the version I was when I was talking to you," she said. "And when I left your office after our session, the cab driver who came to pick me up asked, 'Where to?' 'Home' felt like the wrong answer because I knew home was where the drugs were. So I asked him to take me to the hospital instead. That began my journey of sobriety. Answering those detailed questions with you ignited something in me that I didn't know was there before."

That woman stayed clean for at least two years. I know because I talked to her daughters at that time, and they said she had maintained sobriety.

Remember and believe in the power of description. As your clients co-construct the details of their desired outcome and deeply imagine the difference it will make in their lives, they trigger lasting change. They transform.

Language Creates Reality

A Closer Look with Adam

To add to what Elliott just shared, the session is the intervention because the client's language becomes tangible, and that tangibility becomes real. Furthermore, if you take the notion seriously that language creates reality, then you need to also recognize that change is indeed happening as the client describes it during an SFBT session.

From a neuroscience perspective, this can be described as neuroplasticity. Human brains are always changing and creating synaptic connections from moment to moment. That, in turn, affects the way people experience and make sense of life events, relationships, and themselves. And because people are always changing, it's important to hold on to the fact that SFBT conversations are also creating change—and in a very powerful way. The clients who walk into your office are different from the clients who walk out. With that at the forefront of your mind, you need to be very purposeful about what kind of change you want to create.

If you take the stance we maintain in this approach to honor clients' agency, then the change you create should be consistent with the desired outcome they have established.

At the prompting of your questions, your clients will spend the majority of each session describing the day that change happens, what it will look like, what will be different about themselves when it occurs, how they will act, what they will think, what they will eat, what their partner will notice, what their co-workers will notice, what their friends will notice, what their children will notice, what their pet will notice, etc.

As they describe detail after detail about the change being present, their brains will begin to change, and that change will become reality. It happens by talking about change, thinking about change, conversing about change.

That's why you don't have to do anything beyond conducting a description conversation in order for your clients to be different when they leave your office. That's why the session in and of itself is the intervention. Your work has been done, and it's been done simply by asking your clients to describe the day when the version of themselves that they hope to transform into is present.

Future-Focused Present Tense

A Closer Look with Adam

One aspect that might be an indication that change is happening during the preferred-future conversation is when the client's language changes tense. This isn't something you need to try to control or cause to happen, but it is often a quiet indication that the conversation is creating change.

When you co-construct a preferred-future description, you ask question after question about the presence of their desired outcome. Your clients may struggle to answer at first, but over the course of a session, what most often happens is that the conversation becomes smoother and picks up pace. Your clients will stop imagining their desired outcome and instead start living it. They'll answer questions before you finish asking them. They'll talk as if suddenly they know every answer without thinking, and they'll share them in a rapid-fire way.

Oftentimes, they even switch from talking in future-tense language to present-tense language. Instead of "I would do this," they say, "I *do* this." They're now truly in the moment of their new reality. From that pivot point, the entire conversation shifts to a language I call "future-focused present tense." Through it, the preferred-future conversation is no longer about describing a day when change occurs; it's about *today*. That word, *today*, even slips into the conversation.

The momentum that builds between the therapist and client doesn't happen organically. It happens because you, the therapist, are consistently applying the principles of co-construction: listening to your clients' language and implementing their words, honoring their agency as they express it through their language, and applying your expertise in structuring the session around their desired outcome.

It's up to you to create an environment where your clients can thrive in this process. Over time, as you continue to embed greatness in your questions and as you take a future-focused present tense stance about your clients—asking them to see what's possible but talking to them as if it's happening right now—your clients will get on board. They'll build confidence in you as you build confidence in them.

This isn't manipulation on your part; it's belief. When you view your clients as capable, they also start viewing themselves in that way. The momentum builds until they live life in the full power of their capability.

Chapter 17

History of the Outcome

A Diamond Description Pathway

The Discovery of Exceptions

Around 1978, after Steve de Shazer and Insoo Kim Berg co-founded the Brief Family Therapy Center in Milwaukee, they set out in search of "the perfect client" to test their ideas on. Here's how Elliott remembers that story as told to him by Chris Iveson.

The perfect client needed to be a really difficult client, someone who had a "perfect problem," meaning it was constantly present in that person's life. If Steve and Insoo could figure out a way to solve the perfect client's problem, they could prove that their new approach was successful.

In response to their search, they got a referral from a prominent psychiatric hospital for a woman who struggled with agoraphobia. This woman hadn't left her home in four years. Steve was elated. He had found the perfect client!

When he went to her apartment to meet her, she hesitantly answered the door, yanked him inside, slammed the door, and locked several locks behind her. Steve attempted to conduct a solution focused session that went very poorly, and she ended up yelling, "Get out!"

Dejected, Steve went back to his office and discussed what had happened with Insoo. Knowing she was better with people, she said she would go with Steve a second time to visit this woman. Maybe they'd have better luck.

They knocked on the door of the perfect client's apartment, but no one answered this time. They didn't know what to do or even think. Was the woman with agoraphobia really not at home?

As they puzzled over the situation, the woman suddenly came running toward them from the opposite end of the apartment building hallway, two young children in tow. She rushed past Steve and Insoo, who were waiting by her front door. She unlocked the door, pulled the young children into the apartment, yanked Steve and Insoo inside as well, and locked the several locks behind her.

Steve and Insoo were completely dumbfounded. Insoo said to the woman, "I don't understand. I was told you hadn't left your apartment in four years."

"Well, I don't leave my house except for when my sister can't pick up my children from the bus stop," the woman explained.

"How often is that?" Steve asked.

"About once a week."

Steve and Insoo felt deflated. Their perfect client wasn't so perfect after all. Her problem wasn't consistent. It didn't happen once a week when she had to pick up her kids, even if she didn't view that deviation as a choice or a reprieve from her agoraphobia.

Steve and Insoo soon realized there was no such thing as the perfect client or the perfect problem. Instead, there are always exceptions, times when the problem isn't happening or is happening less often. Even the woman with agoraphobia, who hadn't left her home in four years, had a weekly exception to her problem.

This discovery of exceptions proved to be revolutionary, and it led to the first difference between the MRI in Palo Alto, California, and Steve and Insoo's "MRI of the Midwest."

As modern-day therapists, we're grateful for the pioneering work that Steve and Insoo brought into our field over 40 years ago. We wouldn't be where we are without them. But as SFBT research continues to grow and we gain more mastery in practicing it, we believe our thinking should also evolve about exceptions. In this chapter we'll explain just how we've done that through the description pathway of history of the outcome.

The Discovery of Instances

In the 1990s at BRIEF in London, Chris Iveson, Harvey Ratner, and Evan George embraced the idea of exceptions and used it in their work for a decade until they made their own realization: Maybe exceptions weren't only times when the problem is gone or less frequent. Maybe the outcome is also present.

To put this into context, think of the woman who didn't experience agoraphobia when she picked up her children from the bus stop. Instead of identifying that as an exception, perhaps it could be described as a time when her desired outcome was present because she was able to leave her apartment. The BRIEF therapists began to call these occurrences *instances*, meaning instances of the outcome being present rather than merely exceptions to the problem.

Earlier in this book, we discussed SFBT 1.0 vs. 2.0. Along with the use of presuppositions, another big difference between these two evolutions of the approach is the identification of instances.

The Discovery of History of the Outcome

The solution focused approach continued to evolve in our work as we expanded upon the ideas of exceptions and instances. As we started to analyze the importance of the outcome being present in SFBT conversations, we realized that if A is true (there are always exceptions to problems), and B is true (the outcome is present in instances of those exceptions), then C must also be true (there is a history of that outcome).

Regarding the woman with agoraphobia, exceptions to her problem happened when she was able to leave her apartment, which were instances when her outcome was present. And because those exceptions and instances were true, then her history of the ability to do that could be examined. We do that through the history-of-the-outcome description pathway on the diamond.

As the therapist, you can look back in the timeline of your clients' lives and examine when their outcome showed up. You can ask questions such as:

- How did you help the outcome show up?
- What did you notice when the outcome showed up?
- What difference did it make to you when the outcome showed up?
- What difference did it make to your partner/friend/parent/co-worker when the outcome showed up?

The options are endless.

Let's say you're working with a couple and you ask, "What are your best hopes from our talking?"

"We'd like to be happy again," they answer.

Couples often insert the word *again*, which should alert you to the fact that they're aware that their outcome—in this case, being happy—has a history of being present in their lives. And you can ask them about that history:

- When you were happy last time, how did you notice it?
- What were the clues?
- When was it present?
- What difference did it make to you?
- What difference did it make to your partner?

You could spend an entire session reviewing the history of the outcome. There is so much richness in noticing in the past.

One of the things SFBT gets criticized for is that it only looks at the future, but much of where success and confidence come from—much of what will help our clients reach their desired outcome—are the things they've already done in the past.

As you spend time asking your clients about those things, you're going to get information that will help them pivot and look forward. You can then ask, "If you keep doing those things, or if those things happened again, what would you notice?"

Clients often take for granted the moments that their outcome is present. They say things like, "Ninety-nine percent of the time I deal with this problem, and I want that to be less." They minimize that one percent of the time. "I guess I'm happy sometimes," they relent, "but not very often."

Remember that SFBT is a difference-led approach, so be sure to highlight difference through the questions you ask such as, "Can you tell me about that one percent of the time that's different for you?"

Sometimes clients claim that they've never been happy, they've never gotten along with their partner, they've never been confident, but again remember that if people say they want something, it means they must have at least sampled it at some point in their lives.

When your clients tell you they have a problem, that problem will always have an exception. Think about it in this context: if you had a headache your entire life from the moment you were born until today, how would you know you had a headache? There must have been a moment when the headache disappeared or reduced in intensity that let you know it was solvable and therefore a problem. If it never disappeared or reduced in intensity, you wouldn't know you had a problem.

Count on the fact that there will be an exception whenever clients say *never*. *Always* and *never* are words that should immediately tip you off to remember the rule of exceptions and from there be able to examine the history of the outcome.

The Reverse-Miracle Question

History-of-the-outcome questions can be thought of as "reverse-miracle questions." If you recall from the preferred-future chapter, the miracle question refers to asking clients about the presence of their desired outcome in their future.

If you are working with a client who wants to feel peace, you could ask the miracle question by saying something like, "Suppose you woke up tomorrow and felt peace. What would you notice?" The miracle question is always about the future—most often a future that happens tomorrow.

The reverse-miracle question is similar, but it's about the client's past. For example, "When peace showed up in the past, how did you notice it?"

So the miracle question is a "How *would* you notice it?" question, and the reverse-miracle question is a "How *did* you notice it *in the past*?" question.

The reverse-miracle question is a way—though not the only way—to begin a conversation about the history of the outcome. You can go from the initial question, "So when peace showed up in the past, how did you notice it was there?" to questions like, "How did the people around you notice you were feeling peaceful?" and "What difference did that peace make in your life?"

You can ask countless "How did you notice?" questions and extrapolate the same level of detail about the past as you would if you were examining the future.

For years, people viewed solution focused brief therapy as a future-oriented approach, but it's not limited to the future. It's a detail-oriented approach. It's a difference-oriented approach. It's an approach about the outcome that your clients are in pursuit of, and that outcome showing up in their lives and what impact it would have on them.

That's why you need to develop the skill of asking clients about their tomorrow—when their outcome becomes their reality—but you also need to be able to ask them about their past, when their outcome was their reality. And the reverse-miracle question is a great way to begin that conversation.

Helping Clients Identify Their Accountability of Success

A Closer Look with Adam

There's a connection between the description pathways of resource talk and history of the outcome, and that point of connection is what I call accountability.

In resource talk, you essentially ask your clients, "What resources do you have?" and "How do you do those things?" and "How do those resources show up?"

Likewise, in history of the outcome, in some sense you're asking, "What strengths, abilities, and resources do you have?" but you're also asking, "How did you use those resources to bring about this instance?" You're making your clients completely accountable for their success, because they must have done something—used some skills or abilities—to bring about the instance.

Clients might be confused at first and say things like, "I don't really understand what you mean." The language might get a little jumbled, and they may struggle to answer your questions. They'll often say, "I don't think I did anything to make that come about. I'm pretty sure it just happened."

Remember to presuppose the best in them. One of the presuppositions we maintain in this approach is believing that clients *had* to contribute something to bring about their past instances. Those outcomes didn't just happen by chance.

Clients say, "I don't know, I don't know, I don't know," but as you keep asking and rephrasing your questions, they will start to bring up more details in the description. Elliott and I have found that when clients are asked about what the experience of a solution focused session was like, they answer, "I remembered things I didn't know that I remembered."

Through research, we know that positive emotion and its impact expands a person's vision—not just current or creative vision but also memory vision (Madan, Scott, & Kensinger, 2019). People start to remember more than they knew that they remembered.

So be patient and persistent as they think through and try to articulate their answers, because doing so takes a lot of effort. Help them focus on how they contributed to difference. What really happened that made their best hopes show up?

Together, once you take the time to examine those instances and identify what made your clients accountable for them, you can easily pivot to the present by saying, "Suppose you use that same skill again, or suppose you got those circumstances to be just right again, what would let you know that this instance started showing up in your life once more? What would be different?"

Remember, people tend to take their greatness for granted. They often have a long history of the problem, so sometimes they overlook the history of success. As a result, they might not catch those instances of success when they happen again.

It's your job to help open their eyes. You can do that by asking them to describe, "If that success came back, how would you know? What would you notice?"

History of the Outcome in Couples Therapy

Diving Deep with Elliott

Each partner in a couple lives with their greatest instance—the greatest history of their best hopes being present—and that is that they chose to get together. There was a time when they got along and liked each other and thought the other was attractive. But couples rarely take accountability for the history of their outcome. They forget why they entered into their relationships and how they once worked together to build upon what each had to offer.

As a therapist, you need to give them complete accountability for that success. My favorite question to transition to a history-of-the-outcome conversation with couples is, "How did you meet?"

Let's say a married couple has come to therapy and the wife is super mad. If I was to ask the mad version of the wife, "What do you like about your husband?" the answer I'd likely get is, "Nothing!" But the most beautiful thing about doing a history-of-the-outcome description with couples is that it often cools the emotional temperature in the room.

Imagine instead that I asked the wife, "I can see that you're really angry, but can you tell me how you met your husband?" That question would help her think of something different, something better. She can't describe the experience of meeting her partner, even if she's upset with him, without getting in touch with the feelings and emotions she had when they first met. It's just how human brains work.

By asking that "how you met" question, for the rest of the session I'm no longer talking to the angry version of the wife; I'm talking to a different version, the version that's tapped into the outcome she desires—the outcome she can now relive from her past.

If couples can start describing the influence they had on each other, it moves them to action—to behavior. As they describe the history of the outcome, they begin to act consistently with their best hopes.

You Can't Crave Something You Haven't Sampled

Diving Deep with Elliott

I'm often asked, "What if the client hasn't had a past experience of a desired outcome?" There is no such thing. As I've mentioned several times in this book, if people say that they want something, it means they've at least had a sample of it at some point in the past. People cannot crave or yearn for something that they haven't touched.

To really help this idea hit home, let me tell you about my first visit to New Zealand. After day one of teaching at a conference in Christchurch, the wonderful woman who was hosting me asked what I would like for dinner. She knew that when I travel, I like to try foods that I can't get easily back home in Texas, so she introduced me to a popular New Zealand food that I'd never heard of before called *kebabs*.

Kebabs are different from what we refer to as kabobs in the United States, which are more like a skewer with meat and vegetables. Instead, this kebab was like a big wrap filled with sauce and meat and yogurt and whatever I requested to put inside. When I took a bite, it was utterly delicious and glorious.

Now if Adam were to say to me, "Elliott, what do you want to eat today?" I now have a file folder in my head for "kebab." I can now answer, "I would really like to find a kebab shop." I couldn't have done that before because I had no file folder for it, no access point. So anytime anyone tells you they want something, it means they've had at least a little bit of it in the past, even if they can't recall it.

In order to do solution focused brief therapy well, you have to master the ability to believe in people and not just take their statements at face value, because people's words often violate their truth. If a client tells me, "I've never felt happiness before," I've had to train my brain to not believe that. Because in order to live a life with absolutely no happiness, this client would never have laughed, never have joked, never have smiled. People talk in absolutes when they really don't mean absolutely.

Again, every time your clients tell you they want something, that's your evidence that they've had it before, and you then have the opportunity to co-construct a history-of-the-outcome description with them. You can start by asking a question like, "When happiness showed up in your life before, how did you notice it?"

Utilize presuppositions to trust that your clients have at least had a sampling of the outcome in the past to want to crave it again.

History-of-the-Outcome Example with Laura

Let's return to Elliott's client, Laura, who has a nonverbal son with a severe brain injury. The first thing she answered when Elliott asked her the best-hopes question was, "I want to hear my son call me *Mom*."

In the session, Elliott next asked her about the difference that hearing her son call her *Mom* would make, which led Laura to establish her desired outcome of wanting to be a normal mom.

But what if Elliott hadn't done the work to establish that realistic desired outcome? What if he made a big mistake that many SFBT therapists make, and he used Laura's first response—wanting to hear her son call her *Mom*—to launch into a discussion about exceptions? In that scenario, he would have asked her, "So has there been a time that your son called you *Mom*?"

As you can imagine, Laura's response would have been a devastating, "No," and Elliott would feel terrible too. He would have just introduced sadness into the session, which is the opposite of the hopeful experience he's striving for.

This is why it's so important to center the conversation around a meaningful and realistic desired outcome. Elliott was able to use the realistic outcome—feeling like a normal mom—when he began his history-of-the-outcome description with Laura.

Elliott: Can you tell me about a time when you felt like a normal mom with your son?

Laura: Well, when he was a newborn and I was kind of still completely dazed and confused about what was going on, he was just still to me like a normal newborn baby. So for the first three months, there were a few things that weren't quite normal, but mostly I felt pretty normal then.

Notice that Elliott asked Laura about more than just the exception, because exceptions are identified as times when the problem is either gone or dissipated. Instead, he asked her about the history of the outcome—when the outcome was present in the past—and she was able to share beautiful examples, which gave Elliott the opportunity to ask her more questions about those experiences and co-construct a rich description with her.

Elliott: If I had a chance to meet you when your son was an infant and you were feeling like a normal mom, what would you have told me that you were noticing then that gave you a clue that this normal mom feeling was present?

Laura: Well, I was deliriously happy back then because I just completely decided that all the doctors were wrong because my son looked normal to me. So I was like, "Oh, they've clearly made a mistake." I mean, that shattered quickly enough, but for those three months I was just super happy being at home with my baby and just getting on with life.

Elliott: And what did you notice about yourself that told you you were happy? How did you notice the happiness being present?

Laura: Actually, the pinnacle moment of when I felt like a normal mom was when he smiled for the first time. He couldn't make any sound initially because he'd had breathing tubes, so his vocal cords were damaged and he couldn't even cry—which didn't last. And when he was about seven weeks old, he smiled for the first time, and that seemed so normal. And for me as a mom, it was the best thing. I thought, *It doesn't matter what happens after this because I know that he can show me he's happy.* And so I felt like now I had what I needed to know how to meet his needs, because he could tell me he was happy, and he could tell me he wasn't.

Elliott: So once you knew he could communicate that he was happy or he wasn't happy, that made a difference?

Laura: Yeah, and for me to know that he could experience happiness and joy was really important. That almost, like, set the feeling of "He can have some kind of quality of life, whatever the outcome is," like if he can show me he's happy, he can experience happiness, and that was a major big thing for me. And it felt like a normal mom thing to be in your baby's face, completely annoyingly like you do with a newborn baby until you get a smile, getting a "face ache" when you're trying to make them smile.

Elliott: A face ache? I've never heard of that.

Laura: Yeah, when you're so in their face with your big smiley face, trying to get them to smile back. And you do it so much that your cheeks ache.

Elliott: Once you noticed this normal thing in your son, what did you notice about yourself that triggered a normal mom feeling for you?

Laura: Well, I think that I was fortunate enough that I had two children before him, so I recognized the experience of getting a first smile and those early smiles, so I recognized the magic that that is. And it was more magical because I didn't expect it to happen with my [nonverbal] son.

Elliott: What difference did this magic make to you?

Laura: It just kind of gave me a sense that everything would be okay. I mean, I didn't know what that meant, but for my son to be able to be responsive enough to smile at me appropriately, that made me feel—if I'm relating it to feeling like a normal mom—I guess it's just like an unspoken connection, and that connection has remained for fifteen years. I can still get in his face just like he's still a wee baby, and he will appropriately smile like you would expect.

Again, note that Elliott wasn't asking questions about exceptions; he was asking questions about the history of the presence of the outcome, which in this case was about the presence of Laura feeling like a normal mom while interacting with her nonverbal son. Did you catch how Elliott helped her turn that history of the outcome into a description? It would have been very hard for him to turn an exception into a description.

From the moment Laura told Elliott, "I want to feel like a normal mom," he knew she must have felt like a normal mom at some point in her life. That allowed him to ask, "Can you tell me about a time when you felt like a normal mom with your son?" And as it turned out, against all odds, Laura had experienced that feeling when her son was an infant, and a piece of it persisted to this day.

So in order to be able to follow the history-of-the-outcome description pathway, you have to accept that when your clients say they want something (their desired outcome), that is evidence that they must have had at least a piece of it in the past.

Maintain faith and belief in your clients. Presuppose the best in them and trust in their capability. If Elliott hadn't believed that Laura had ever felt like a normal mom before, he couldn't have asked her to describe a time when she had experienced that outcome. Faith and belief come first.

Once you believe that your clients' desired outcome is real, then it must be real in the future, and there must be evidence of it in the past. And as it turned out, there were touching examples of Laura feeling like a normal mom in her past.

Descriptions have the same impact whether they're about tomorrow (the preferred future) or looking backward (the history of the outcome) because it's the details of the outcome that are transformative, not the timeline of those details.

Facing Cancer by Drawing Upon the History of the Outcome

A Closer Look with Adam

As I mentioned in an earlier chapter, in May 2019 my wife was diagnosed with breast cancer. I found out when I was out of state with Elliott—we were teaching at an event in Florida. After my wife had a routine doctor's appointment, she called and said, "They're doing more tests, and I'm not quite sure what it means."

"Do you need me to come home?" I asked, concerned.

"No, I think I'll be okay," she said. "I'll call you when I get the results."

Nervous, I went back to where I was teaching with Elliott. "At some point I'm going to get a phone call," I told him, "and I'll need to step out."

Soon enough, my phone rang in my pocket, and I left the room again.

When I answered the phone, my wife was crying. I knew whatever test results she had received weren't good.

"What's going on?" I asked.

"I got diagnosed with breast cancer," she said.

My mind started to race. How could this be happening? What would happen to *her*? As I stood there for a minute, taking in the news, the only thing I could come up with to say to her was, "How do you know that, no matter what happens, you're going to be okay?" And by *going to be okay*, I didn't even mean that she was going to live. I just meant that she would be okay as she went through the process of battling cancer.

My wife cried for a bit more and then paused to compose herself before she said the most profound thing I believe anyone could say in that moment. "Because I've done hard things before," she said.

We spent about a half an hour talking about the hard things that she in particular had been through, and how we had been okay through those times.

After that phone call, I went back into the room where I had been teaching with Elliott. He looked at me anxiously and gave me a thumbs-up, but I had to give him a thumbs-down. His shoulders fell. He knew that the outcome wasn't what we were hoping for.

The time came for my wife to undergo surgery in order to have the cancer removed. Afterward, she and I drove our kids from Georgia to Virginia, where my sister lives. My sister had offered to watch our kids for a while so my wife and I could spend some time together and focus on starting chemotherapy.

After we dropped off our kids, we embarked on our drive back to Georgia. During those nine hours, we revisited the idea of "You've done hard things before."

I said, "Knowing tomorrow that you have to do your first round of chemotherapy, and not knowing what that's going to be like, what do you know about yourself that lets you know you can do this hard thing? What have you learned about yourself, as you have dealt with other hard things, that you are glad you know going into this hard thing? What will tell you that you are using that knowledge and those qualities about yourself this time?"

We went back in time and talked about the really hard things we had done before and in the context of how we overcame them.

What skills did we use to make it through? Who were the helpful people around us who contributed to helping us accomplish and endure those really hard things? In essence, we were doing a blend of history of the outcome and resource talk.

We talked about the two times my wife had experienced miscarriages, and how one of those miscarriages happened on Mother's Day. We talked about the women who had reached out to my wife, women who had also experienced miscarriages. They rallied around her and supported her and shared how they had recovered. Family members also came to spend time with us and helped us keep going.

My wife and I also talked about how, at that point in our lives, we had moved across the country three different times in our marriage. We talked about how hard it was to leave our families and friends and support systems, and how in each of the moves, we were going to a place we had never been to before.

Again, we talked about those hard times in the context of how we endured and overcame them. We remembered how our church community supported us and how financial help was also given.

Over this nine-hour conversation, we realized that, although those times in the past were difficult, in the end they didn't drag us down. They weren't too hard to overcome. Instead, they were experiences that made us stronger, events that held us together, ways we learned about ourselves, times we discovered who we were.

We realized we could take all that strength with us as we faced this new challenge in our lives. We could bring all the people, the networks, the experiences, and the memories.

That conversation was like an anchor to us throughout the nine months of treatments that Becca endured. On the particularly hard days, we would reflect on what we were learning this time that we wanted to make sure we didn't forget. On the particularly good days, we made sure to be extra grateful for the smallest moments of relief. On days where support came from individuals bringing us dinner, sending flowers and cards, or calling with messages of support, we made sure to take note that our support system was rallying around us again.

Because we had taken time to think about our history of managing hard things, we were so much more aware when history repeated itself in the best ways possible. That's the real power of having a history-of-the-outcome conversation.

Outcomes Don't Necessarily Need to Directly Correlate

As a therapist, whenever a client establishes what they truly want, you have to remember that they've done hard things before, they've managed difficulty, and they've overcome challenges. Through SFBT, we highlight strength, ability, capability. We hold the stance of believing in people and seeing them as powerful.

Your clients' history of the outcome doesn't necessarily have to translate into the word-for-word desired outcome that they say they want. Adam's wife had never been diagnosed with breast cancer before, but she had done other hard things from which she could draw lessons.

Let's say you have a client named David who says, "I want to be happy in my work environment." You don't have to begin a history-of-the-outcome description by asking a question like, "When were you the most happy in your job?" You could also ask, "When were you the most happy in your life?"

Maybe David was the most happy when he was a five-year-old kid and didn't have a job. You can still draw on that description of a happy kid and ask, "If those things returned and you incorporated them into being a happy employee, how would you notice that those things were back in your life?"

Legacy Questions

By now, you've probably realized how important the past is in SFBT. Every human being on the planet has a hero in the history of their own life's story. So to only focus on the future in solution focused brief therapy is to ignore that hero. As a therapist, you need to be skilled in asking about people's yesterdays because that's where their hero is. And every single person has been influenced by someone, and that influence is in the past.

In 2021, we spent two weeks on a trip visiting prominent places associated with the civil rights movement, where we interviewed several people. We learned that an entire generation of civil rights leaders, including Medgar Evers and Martin Luther King, Jr., were inspired—and we use that word sensitively—by the death of Emmett Till.

Everybody has been influenced by someone, and through exploring the history of the outcome, you can help your clients tap into those influences. One of our favorite ways to do that is to ask what we call "legacy questions."

A legacy is when your clients were at their peak and when they're desired outcome was present. Legacy questions reveal what actions they took to make it present, and the qualities and characteristics they drew upon to make the desired outcome possible.

As we mentioned in Chapter 10, the legacy conversation is another place where history of the outcome intersects with resource talk. On the one hand, you're asking, "Where did you get that resource?" but you're also asking about it in the context of how that resource—that legacy—was handed off to your clients in the past. Here are some examples of legacy questions:

- Where did you learn to be brave?
- Where did you learn that you were the kind of person who was capable of being happy?
- Who helped you realize that you had what it took to be confident?
- What was that like?
- How did that process happen?
- How did you know you were receiving it?
- What did it mean to you when that person handed this legacy off to you?
- How did you let them know you were pleased that you had inherited this legacy?

By asking clients questions about where their legacy came from, they oftentimes introduce you to the most important people in their lives—people who changed them for the better. Meeting those people, even through conversation, becomes an honor. Discuss them with respect and care.

After meeting them, you can then ask, "And if somehow that person could see you now, what would they notice to let you know that you're carrying that legacy on in just the right way?" or "What do they see in you that lets them know you're holding their legacy with honor?"

There's so much power that can come through talking about the past, and oftentimes it's something that solution focused therapists forget to bring into their sessions or they get critiqued for forgetting.

Practice history-of-the-outcome and legacy questions by asking people, "Think about the time in your life when you were at your very best." From there, ask them to describe themselves at that time in their life. What was different when they were at their best? How did they get to be their best? Then shift into legacy questions by asking, "Where did that legacy come from?"

How to Ask Legacy Questions

Before you transition into a legacy-questions conversation, it's often helpful to ask your clients to identify an important resource. Consider the following excerpt from a session Adam conducted with Janie, who is an author of creative fiction and who struggles with depression.

Adam: What is a characteristic, skill, or trait that you have that you are most proud of?

Janie: Probably writing.

Adam: And what characteristic do you have inside of you that shows you're a good writer?

Janie: Well, I think I share truth, even though it's fiction.

Adam: How do you ensure that you're telling your story with a filter of truth?

Janie: If I can just focus on writing for me—writing something I will enjoy and that I find good and entertaining—then that ensures that the truth is there. I have to make it personal.

Adam: And what do you call that quality that it has to be good and personal?

Janie: I don't know if it has a word.

Adam: If you somehow came up with the right word, what would you call it?

Janie: Say the question again?

Adam: When you say, "I'm being true to me and that shows up in my writing," what is it called when you're being true to you?

Janie: Authenticity.

Notice that Adam persisted until Janie answered with the word for her specific resource—in this case, the characteristic of authenticity. Adam needed her word, not a word he could have come up with on his own. Once he had Janie's word, he could transition from talking about resources to a legacy-questions conversation.

Adam: Who taught you that authenticity was something you should value?

Janie: My dad, because he was a writer.

Adam: And how did you learn from him that authenticity was something that you could and should value?

Janie: He was just born artistic, but his dad was not that way. He had this real struggle with his dad and had to pave the way on his own to know it was okay to choose the artist's life. I saw him pay lots of sacrifices for that life because he was often self-employed and there were highs and lows in his career. But he wouldn't change that because he was being true to himself. I was also his child who just kind of naturally picked up on writing, even though I didn't identify myself as a writer until my thirties because I pursued acting for a long time. But he showed me from a very young age that he valued my artistic opinion. I think it's because he could tell I was an artist, even though he wasn't trying to mold me into a writer. And I think he didn't want to be like his dad. He wanted to show me that it was okay to be an artist.

Adam: How did he communicate that he saw the artist in you, but that it was okay for you to be an actor and not a writer? How did he communicate that you could be your own kind of artist?

Janie: Like the things he did or the words he said?

Adam: Either.

Janie: It was more just how he showed it to me. He got excited when he could help me with creative writing papers for school. He came to all my plays. But I think above all, the thing that I remember from a very young age was just that he respected my artistic opinion. For a while, he was a publisher of music and books, and he would ask me, "What do you think about this cover? What do you think about this music? What do you think about this story?" And he honestly valued my opinion, because he would make changes based on what I said from a very young age.

Adam: In those moments when he would listen to you, when he would value your opinion and would make changes, how did you let him know you were pleased that he valued your artistic opinion?

Janie: I remember just beaming. Once he invited me into a room where other adults were looking at these pictures for a product they were making. And I said what I thought about one of them, and in front of everyone, my dad said, "Wow, Janie's right. That picture looks better when the orientation is flipped." So I remember just feeling like a beaming feeling.

Then, as I got older, whenever he'd ask for my input, I'd be really excited and set aside anything else I was doing for an hour and talk with him about the plot of his book or whatever he wanted my feedback on. I remember being just as excited as he conveyed that he was also excited to talk together.

Adam: And as you think back on those moments where you set aside all the things that you had going on and spent that hour with him, what difference do you think that made for him?

Janie: Well, since I was such an artistic child, I think we had a bond that way. And even though I didn't think about it like this until now, it was probably just as validating for him as it was for me. I feel like my dad and I really understood each other.

Adam: And what difference does it make to you to realize that you were, through that bond and connection, giving him validation while he was giving you validation?

Janie: What difference does it make to me? That's a strangely hard question.

Adam: I know. It is hard.

Janie: I just felt seen, and I just really wanted to please him. He would have been proud of me anyway, but I really wanted to make him proud.

Adam: If you could make him proud in a way that is completely authentic to you, what would be the most appropriate way to make him proud while staying true to who you are?

Janie: Well, he unexpectedly passed away a few years ago, so I think the main thing I try to carry with me is that I need to believe in myself as much as he believed in me. Because here I am in the artist's life, and there are highs and lows. So no matter how the tide rolls, I have to just believe in myself.

Adam: What does it mean to you that you can ride the tide like your dad did, and throughout all the highs and lows that you hold on to the belief he had in you that you can do it? What does it mean to you that you get to hold on to that vision?

Janie: I feel like I'm carrying his legacy forward. That I can continue to give what he was giving to the world.

That's the essence of a legacy-questions conversation. Once Adam arrived at Janie's word, *authenticity*, and once she identified the person whom she learned that from, he spent the rest of the description asking her questions like, "How did your dad teach you to be authentic?" and "How did you show him you were glad that he was teaching you to be authentic?" and "Now that you've gained this vision of authenticity, how do you carry it forward?" and "What does it mean that you get to be authentic in that way?"

So Janie's legacy is authenticity, but the questions are about how she learned it, how her dad taught it to her, and how she showed him she was grateful for it. In essence, the questions were about the difference that it made to her to receive authenticity from her dad.

The really powerful thing about a history-of-the-outcome description (and in this case, doing legacy questions) is that, even though your clients are talking about something that happened in their past, they're now more likely to think about how it applies to their present and future. In other words, it impacts what they do now, and it causes them to transform.

Chapter 18

Closing the Session

The Bottom Point of the Diamond

The Gift Shop of the Anne Frank House

Diving Deep with Elliott

A few years ago, Chris Iveson and I found ourselves in Amsterdam. As luck would have it, we were both teaching at separate SFBT events that were taking place within two blocks of each other. Being the good friends that we are, we arranged to go out to dinner.

To pass the time until our reservation at a nearby restaurant, we went for a walk. It was a cold and snowy January day, and our street ran alongside one of the city canals. Along that street, we came across a building with a sign that read, "Anne Frank Huis" (Anne Frank House).

I turned to Chris and asked, "Is this *the* Anne Frank House?"

"I don't know," he said.

"How long have you been coming to Amsterdam?" I asked.

"Thirty years."

"And you've never gone in here?"

He looked a little sheepish. "No."

"Well, I want to go into the Anne Frank House," I said.

We walked inside, paid the fee, and started the tour. We passed through a hallway, turned the corner, and came across a bookcase that was halfway open. Behind the bookshelf was a hidden staircase. The tour guide let us know that this was the access point to the annex where Anne Frank had stayed while she lived in hiding during World War II.

In respectful silence, Chris and I explored that annex. An excerpt from Anne's diary was displayed on one of the walls. Another wall had pencil marks that measured how tall she had grown while she stayed there. Everything was deeply touching.

We went down another set of stairs as we left the annex, and there was a picture on the wall of Anne Frank with her elementary school class and teacher. Each student was numbered, and there was a key beside the picture that explained what later happened to each individual. Written on it were things like, "Student 1 died at such and such concentration camp. Student 2 died at such and such concentration camp." By this point, Chris and I were in tears and holding on to each other for support.

At the end of the tour, we passed through a gift shop in order to exit the house. We stayed in that gift shop for a few seconds, then walked outside, where we finally started talking. The first words we shared were about how moving the experience was and how remarkably well the house had been preserved.

The Nazis had gone into the house and stripped it down, but the one person who still had access to the annex and who survived World War II was Otto Frank, Anne's father, and he restored the annex in the way that it remains today.

My conversation with Chris soon turned to solution focused brief therapy. He said, "The gift shop is kind of like the ending of a solution focused session. There's nothing truly valuable there, and we spend the least amount of time there."

He was right. Everything in the actual museum of the Anne Frank House was priceless. If we were to erase the marks on the wall that measured Anne's height, we would have erased something priceless. There were also magazine pages she had pasted on the wall that were covered by protective glass. All of those things were precious and irreplaceable. In comparison, the items in the gift shop were only cheap replicas.

We had literally spent 2 hours in the museum and only 10 seconds in the gift shop. This became a metaphor for us in how we end an SFBT session. The closing is the least important part of the session, so we simply say, "Good-bye."

That good-bye is composed of a thank you and an invitation to return if the client desires. For example, you could say, "Thank you for answering all my questions. If you'd like another session, I'd be happy to meet with you again. Thanks for coming."

You don't need to do anything more, because the conversation itself is what makes the impact. That's how this approach works. As Adam consistently says, "The session is the intervention."

By the time you get to the end of the session, you're operating under the assumption that something has come up during that time that has made a difference in the way your clients are going to live their lives. Your job is to simply honor their agency and say something like, "Thank you for answering my questions. I know some of them were difficult, and I appreciate you spending the time to answer them for me. If you think another session would be useful, I'm happy to do that. Have a good day."

That's how we end sessions. And that's why we end them the way we do.

Resist the tendency to become a compliment machine, a feedback machine, or a suggestion robot. Refrain from the urge to make sure your clients change by encouraging them.

Instead, trust their capability and honor their autonomy. Treat them like a helium balloon. A helium balloon does not need any encouragement to float. All you have to do is let it go, and it rises.

When you get to the end of a session, your job is to do just that—let go and don't get in the way of your clients' progress. Let them go like you'd let a balloon go.

Trust That Language Creates Reality

A Closer Look with Adam

Trust that a different version of your client is going to leave your session versus the one who arrived. You do that through language.

If you hold on to that idea that language creates reality, remember that you just spent 50 minutes talking with your clients as they richly described the presence of their desired outcome. Consequently, they're leaving the session in a new reality, and they have to engage with that new reality in a different way.

You don't know what's different about them yet, and they don't know either. They can't know until they go out and engage in the world as a different and transformed person. That's when they'll start to notice, "Oh, that's different about me," and "I wouldn't have done that before," and "Hey, I'm doing that thing again."

In closing the session, you don't want to do anything that could mess up that discovery. Some ways you can mess it up is by saying, "Instead of just going and doing what you're going to do, go do this thing that I want you to do." Those things can be homework or tasks or prescribed interventions. You can also mess up a session by summarizing it or paying compliments. Trust in your clients and do all you can to protect their autonomy.

Never Pay Compliments

Although this topic was already covered on the "Nevers" list in Chapter 5, it is important to reiterate it here, because compliments were historically the premiere topic discussed at the end of SFBT sessions. What we're suggesting is an evolution of the approach and may challenge many SFBT clinicians.

Paying compliments violates your clients' autonomy because clients are handed your impression of them rather than understanding their greatness on their own as they leave your office to make changes.

Resist the urge to say things like, "You know, as you described that for forty-five minutes, there were some things that stood out to me that I thought were particularly important. I was so impressed when you said that one thing, and when you later said that other thing, I was also amazed by you."

Compliments place pressure on your clients because they make them think, *I have to change in this way or think of myself in that way because my therapist told me I was this kind of person.*

Instead, give clients the agency to decide who they have become through the session on their own and to make changes as they see fit.

Never Summarize

We know from research that when you ask therapists versus clients, "What was the most helpful moment of therapy?" they will tell you two different things. Nine times out of ten, what was meaningful to the therapist is different from what was meaningful to the client. That's why you don't want to summarize the session for your clients.

When you summarize, you change what they think is important, because now they consider what you think as more important. You're giving them your perception of the conversation instead of allowing them to have their own understanding.

Again, in SFBT you need to do everything you can to maintain your clients' autonomy, and that means closing the session as simply as possible. For example, "Well, I guess we're out of time. Thanks for coming. Thanks for answering my questions. If you want to come back, you're welcome to." That's it. If you do anything more, you've stepped over the bounds of your role, and you've forced yourself into your clients' role.

Never Assign Homework or Tasks

When solution focused brief therapy first started, Steve de Shazer and Insoo Kim Berg built an entire session around the very end, when they developed tasks. During therapy, their team observed from behind a one-way mirror and looked for insights on what those tasks needed to be.

Around the 40-minute mark, Steve and Insoo would take a break from the client, leave the room, and go consult with the team. Together, they would come up with a task based on the conversation that had occurred during the session.

Steve and Insoo would then go back to the client and discuss what stood out to the team and what they wanted the client to do between now and the next time they met.

Back then—over 40 years ago—building a session up to assigning a task was a really traditional way to do psychotherapy. And although it wasn't a solution focused perspective, it was what Steve and Insoo had been taught through other approaches.

Fast-forward to today and you'll find that most therapy modalities still teach that we should assign tasks and homework. For instance, many of us were trained in cognitive behavioral therapy (CBT), where we were taught that we needed to tell the client to do something in order to make change happen.

In SFBT we don't believe that. We believe change happens as a consequence of the conversation, because description impacts people. Therefore, we don't need to give clients tasks.

We began to notice that because our clients were different when they left our sessions, they went on to do remarkable things on their own—things that we could never have determined for them.

When they came back and we started the next session by asking, "What's been better?" they would tell us amazing stories, things they had done because they now viewed themselves as different.

Again, we could never have imagined those tasks for them. If anything, we would have set the bar too low. That reinforced our belief that giving our clients a task was also giving them a limitation, which we didn't want to do. We wanted our clients to be limitless, filled with hope, and more armed for change than not.

It all comes back to honoring the client's agency, and a big part of that is allowing our clients the ability to choose whatever they're going to do with this process.

Years ago, when Elliott was a new therapist and practicing CBT, he asked his returning clients, "So how are things going?" They struggled to answer, often saying things like, "I don't remember what we talked about in the previous session" or "I tried to do what we talked about, but it didn't work." There was a constant battle for client compliance.

Once Elliott started practicing solution focused brief therapy, those challenges went away. Clients followed through on their own because now they had buy-in with the process. *They* were the ones providing the answers to questions. They were the ones describing the transformation they desired.

In SFBT, you focus on the outcome that your clients are pursuing. You spend the session asking them, "What would you notice? What would you do? How would you go about that? What things would happen?" You ask them about their perspective, their unique skills and gifts, and their strengths and abilities. You need to honor that work that has happened in the session.

If you get in the way by giving tasks or assigning homework, you're now relying on your own skills and abilities. Resist that tendency. Let your clients make their own choices about what they will or won't do after the session.

We know from experience that that's a scary and nerve-racking thing to do—a thing that many therapists are hesitant to embrace. But it's probably the most important choice we've ever made in our work. Its results are what led us to completely buy into solution focused brief therapy.

Remember that the session itself is the intervention. And if your clients come back to therapy, you'll have the opportunity to ask them, "How did that intervention impact your life?" Their answers will be profound and will blow you away.

Honoring the Client's Free Choice

People often say they love SFBT because it empowers the client, but we struggle with this idea. When most therapists say, "I want to empower the client," what they really mean is, "I want to empower the client as long as the client changes." But the word *autonomy* means free choice, and that includes the choice to *not* benefit from therapy.

At the end of a session, in your desire for your clients to succeed, you might feel the urge to tell them what to do to get better, but that in effect diminishes their agency to choose to get better for themselves.

If you've seen the film *The Matrix*, it's like the choice Neo is given to take the red pill or the blue pill, to choose to free his mind or live in ignorance.

You need to also give your clients that kind of choice. There's something magical about the action of clients choosing to achieve their desired outcome versus them being given the choice to merely comply with what their therapist has told them to do.

Most psychotherapists think their role is to be a helper, and a helper provides education or a task. In an effort to help, they tell their clients what to do. The paradigm shift is the stance that your clients already know what to do. They are the experts in their own lives. And as experts, they will come up with what's most helpful to them.

So honor your clients' autonomy. Honor their agency. Let them be in charge of what they do with their own lives.

Knowing When to Shift from Description to Closing

Beginning SFBT therapists often ask us, "How do you know you've gotten enough details from the description to close the session?"

Our answer is that you have no way of knowing if you've gotten enough details from the description. When to close the session is simply determined by the clock. You get as many details as you can in the time allotted to you, and when that time is up, you're done.

Elliott had a client once who enjoyed the description so much that she asked to have her follow-up sessions be two hours long.

She would make these appointments toward the end of each December, so she and Elliott could meet during the first week of January. During the sessions, she wanted him to ask her, "Suppose we are meeting toward the end of this new year and you're really pleased with the way you conducted yourself over the year. What would you notice?"

She would bring a legal pad, and she'd write down all her answers—her evidence that she was going to have a good year.

So you have no way of knowing what answer makes a difference in your clients' lives. All you can do is co-construct the description with them until the clock tells you that it's time to stop.

Clients Who Are
Mandated to Attend Therapy

Diving Deep with Elliott

You might be wondering how to close a session with clients who are mandated to attend therapy. At an earlier time in my career, I worked with people in this situation, clients who were mandated by court probation to attend a certain number of sessions. At the end of those sessions, I said the same thing to them that I say to my regular clients: "Do you think another session would be useful?"

"Yes," they often replied. "I've still got to come because of my mandate."

But even though they were mandated, they still had the choice to comply with that mandate, and that meant I still needed to respect that choice and honor their agency.

Don't let yourself think that if your clients are mandated, they aren't making a choice. They are—even if the choice is, *Go to therapy or prison.*

Every time I met with clients who were mandated and on probation, I treated them as if they had made the choice to come to see me—because they had.

Q&A about Closing the Session

How do you become comfortable when clients choose to not come back?

First of all, recognize that clients choose not to return after attending *all* types of therapy. That reality isn't exclusive to SFBT. In fact, here's an interesting statistic: across the field of psychotherapy, the modal number of sessions a client attends is one (Dryden, 2018).

As a therapist in general, you need to get used to the fact that your clients may not come back. The brilliance of SFBT is that we maximize the time we have been given with our clients, because the only time we have guaranteed to meet with them is one time—the current session.

Over the course of one month, Elliott worked with a married couple twice. The first session was tremendously impactful, and the second session was a follow-up to that first session. Between that second session and the third that was scheduled, the husband died in a motorcycle accident.

The wife came back to Elliott and said with great emotion, "Thank you for the way you do therapy because I enjoyed life with my husband the last month he was alive. If you had conducted [problem-focused] therapy, where life gets worse before it gets better, we would have been in the 'it gets worse' phase when he passed away. Thank you for bringing out the best in us from the beginning."

Is it okay to ask your clients, "What do you think you'd like to work on between now and the next session?"

No. If you ask that question, you're setting a bar, even though you're asking your clients to set it. You're getting in the way of the description they've done in the session. You need to let them go out into the world and embark on their own exploratory process.

Once you ask, "What do you think you want to work on?" you're removing that creativity and spontaneity and the impact of what happened in the session.

Is it okay to ask your clients, "What impacted you the most about today's session?"

No, because they don't know yet. So much about SFBT is what your clients will notice, but they need time outside of therapy to process the session and enter their changed reality. That's when they'll begin to notice the difference the session made.

In SFBT, we're not interested in, "Do you feel better?" We're interested in, "Are you doing better things?" Your clients can't know the answer to that until they leave, go home, and live their lives.

Resist the urge to ask questions for your own benefit and validation. Trust that you've done a good job by adhering to the tenets of SFBT and not overstepping the bounds of your role.

How do you respond to clients if they say at the end of a session, "Well, that was nice to think about, but how do I actually do it?"

Our usual response to questions like that is, "I don't know, but I look forward to seeing how you figure it out."

PART IV

Beyond the Basics

Chapter 19

Follow-Up Sessions in the Diamond Model

Conducting a Follow-Up Session with Confidence

In solution focused brief therapy, there are two types of sessions: first sessions and all the rest, which are what we call follow-up sessions.

Beginning SFBT therapists often ask us, "What do you do beyond the first session?" This is a common and understandable question since we spend so much time teaching about how to conduct a first session. In this chapter, we'll show you how to conduct any follow-up session with confidence.

No matter if you're in a first session or any session beyond, you'll still follow the three-step process of the diamond: establish a desired outcome, co-construct a description, and close by maintaining the client's autonomy. The diamond always remains your road map.

The only difference between a first session and a follow-up session is that you go into a follow-up session with the knowledge of a desired outcome that you didn't have before you conducted the first session.

You have two choices when your clients return to therapy: you can treat the follow-up session like a first session, or you can ask about your clients' progress.

If we haven't seen a client in several months, we're very likely to say, "I'm glad you're back! So what are your best hopes for today?" Because so much time has passed, we'll just restart the process as if it's the first session again.

But if it's only been a week or two since the first session, we're very likely to start off the conversation by asking, "What's been better?" or "What's been different since we last met?" We'll move forward with the assumption that the client is still interested in the same desired outcome we established from last time.

By asking, "What's been better (or different)?" you go into the session with a presupposition that the client has done things and made changes between this session and the last as a consequence of the last session.

"What's been better?" or "What's been different?" are essentially your way of asking, "So how did it go since the last time I saw you?"

To explore those differences, you can ask history-of-the-outcome questions such as, "How did you notice?" and "What gave you a clue that those differences were happening?" and "Who noticed those differences were happening?"

Or you can ask resource-talk questions like, "How did you make those differences happen?" and "What role did you play?"

If you run out of questions, you can always return to the desired-outcome section of the diamond and ask, "So what are your best hopes for meeting today?" then establish a new desired outcome and co-construct a new description.

Every conversation is different. With some clients, we just ask, "What's been better?" and we spend the entire session reviewing signs of progress. With other clients, we ask, "What's been better?" and we spend only 10 minutes reviewing those signs before we ask for a new desired outcome and restart the process of description.

Follow-up sessions should feel natural. Don't get hung up on any so-called steps of conducting them. Instead of worrying about techniques, we challenge you to think about how to have a solution focused conversation. We want you to become a master conversationalist.

When you do that, it doesn't matter what kind of problem the client comes to therapy with. It doesn't matter how many people are in a session, whether you're working with an individual, a couple, or a family. It doesn't matter if you see children, teens, or adults. And it doesn't matter if you're conducting a first session, a second session, or many sessions beyond.

Once you can be a good conversationalist about desired outcomes, describing the presence of those outcomes, and ending the session in a way that doesn't violate autonomy, then all the other steps and techniques become moot.

Mindset Adjustments about Follow-Up Sessions

A Closer Look with Adam

As a solution focused therapist, you need to shift your thinking about follow-up sessions in a few important ways.

One adjustment I want you to make is to refrain from thinking about a follow-up session as an evaluation of how well you conducted the first session.

If the client comes back and says, "Things are much better," you might interpret that as, "I did a good job last time." But follow-up sessions are not assessment tools. In much of SFBT, we have thrown out assessment tools. We just focus on the business of having meaningful conversations, which is what a follow-up session, like any other session, should be all about.

Another adjustment I recommend is that you don't expect a certain outcome. Just like with the first session, before you establish your clients' best hopes, you don't know how to proceed in a follow-up session until your clients tell you where you're going.

If you begin a follow-up session with an expectation like, *Surely something must be better for my clients*, then you set yourself up to be disappointed. Your clients will recognize that disappointment and respond to it in a way that hinders their progress. At that point, the session is no longer about what they want to get out of therapy; it's about your wish for what they should have done, which is an unfair burden to place on them.

The third adjustment I'd like you to make is to go into a follow-up session thinking, *I'm about to engage in another hopefully useful conversation.* Maintain that mindset whether or not your clients have improved, gotten worse, or stayed the same. It's not your place to judge.

The last adjustment I recommend is that you apply your natural curiosity and conversational skills. Like we mentioned above, follow-up sessions really come down to you being a good conversationalist. Trust in your ability to do this. You have lived your entire life having interactions with people, followed by separations from them, then reunions, during which time you asked questions to catch up on their life.

I do this every weekday with my children. When I send them to school, we are separated for a time; then at the end of the day, when I come home from work and they come home from school, we engage in a conversation in which I ask things like, "How was your day?" and "What was the best part of your day?" and "What things did you do that you particularly liked doing?" Notice how my curiosity is embedded in those questions.

A follow-up SFBT session is similar. You begin the conversation by asking, "What's been better?" which is your way of essentially asking, "How was your time while you were away from me? Can you fill me in?"

If you can go into a follow-up session with no expectations about the outcome but instead genuine curiosity about what occurred while you were apart from your client, you'll find yourself naturally asking those simple kinds of questions.

Take comfort in the fact that you're not going into the session blind. You're armed with presuppositions. For example, when you ask, "What's been better?" you're immediately presupposing change and difference.

Your clients might reply, "Nothing is different. Nothing is better." If so, don't worry. You can bring that answer back to the diamond and ask a resource-talk question such as, "Can you tell me how you managed?"

Strive to find that beautiful balance between presupposing change and not having expectations for what your clients are supposed to do. Even in the simple question, "How was your day?" is the presupposition of "What was the best part?" and "What did you do that you were so pleased with?"

Resist the urge to overthink and apply techniques to force your clients into one avenue of change. Instead, let them tell you what's new and different. Believe in them, follow the outcome they desire, and trust in the process of solution focused brief therapy.

The Three Responses to "What's Been Better?"

Diving Deep with Elliott

There are three ways clients respond when you ask them, "What's been better?"

One, they can say that things are better, in which case I'll likely ask, "How did you contribute to things getting better?" and "What did you notice?"

Two, they can say that things are the same, in which case I'll ask, "How did you keep them the same? What role did you play in the problem not getting worse?" and "How did you notice that things were staying the same?" and "How did you hold on to hope as things were staying the same?"

Or three, clients can say that things are worse. This is the least likely response, but in the rare case it happens, I can ask, "While things were getting worse, how did you show up in a way that pleased you?" and "While things were getting worse, how did you hold on to enough hope to come back to therapy?" and "What did you do to stop things from getting *even* worse?"

Don't believe your clients when they say that nothing has been better, but *believe in* them. When people are in the weeds of a problem, they have a hard time noticing progress.

When a client says nothing's better, another follow-up question that I like to ask is, "So if we had the time between this session and the last session on video, and I watched the whole thing, at what point would I have had the hardest time noticing that nothing was better?" That question really helps the client to consider what has happened for the better since we last met.

No matter the client's response to "What's been better?" you can still craft questions that lead you down a history-of-the-outcome or resource-talk description pathway in a follow-up session.

Chapter 20

The Tool of Scaling

The Benefits of Scaling

Scaling (or "scales") is a conversation tool that includes numeric representations from 0 to 10, in which 10 represents the complete presence of the desired outcome and 0 represents the complete absence of the desired outcome.

Therapists use scales to assist them in the description portion of the diamond. Some people like scales and others don't. Those who do like scales say that they are helpful in the learning process of trying to wrap their heads around SFBT. Scales also facilitated their growth in knowing how to put together questions.

Scales can be thought of as training wheels. They help to give you a format, a structure, for how you go about co-constructing descriptions.

If your client's desired outcome is happiness, you can use a scale to ask, "If you were to move just a little bit closer, maybe half a point up on the scale toward what happiness looks like for you, how would you know? What would you notice?"

Being able to integrate the tool of scaling into your questions is relieving for a lot of therapists. It gives them a sense of confidence, rather than the nerve-racking feeling of "How do I come up with a question to accomplish what I'm trying to accomplish?"

If you choose to use scales, we want you to be endlessly creative with them and keep in mind all the tenets of SFBT as you build questions. Remember to ADOPT the stance, maximize your clients' possibilities, and evoke the best version of them—the version capable of the transformation they desire.

Why Scales Are No Longer in the Diamond Model

Those of you familiar with our work may remember that scaling used to be a description pathway in our first version of the diamond model. We eventually removed scaling from the diamond because we realized it doesn't actually function as a description. Scales are better understood as questions that you can ask to shift between description pathways.

Consider the description pathways of resource talk, preferred future, and history of the outcome. Conversations within those pathways can last for the entirety of a session. But scales are different. They're more of a means to assist you in asking questions along one of those description pathways.

For example, if you're talking about resources, and the client has already established a desired outcome of "I want to be more confident," you can say, "If ten is complete and utter confidence, and zero is the exact opposite of that, where would you say you are now?"

Likewise, if you're in the preferred future, you can say, "How hopeful are you that what we've talked about today can actually come about? Ten is totally hopeful and zero is not hopeful at all." Evan George calls these kinds of scales "hope scales."

Lastly, if you're in the history of the outcome, you can say, "So, when you experienced your desired outcome before, where would you put that on a scale? How did you notice its presence? What was different about that?"

Although you can spend a lot of time doing scales, we don't believe they comprise a description pathway in and of themselves; instead, they typically service another description. In other words, scales are a tool you can use to get a description, but they very rarely stand on their own as a total description mechanism.

We consider scales to be the most helpful when used as a pivot point to steer the conversation in a different direction on the client's timeline.

In our opinion, the most skilled practitioner with scales is Harvey Ratner at BRIEF in London. We've studied Harvey's work for years, and he'll say things to his clients like, "Can I do a scale?" The client will say, "Sure." He'll then ask, "If ten represents that you're happy and the person you'd like to be, and zero is the exact opposite, where are you today?" The client will say a number such as, "I'm at a three."

At that point, Harvey has a choice to make about where to pivot the conversation. He can say, "Suppose tomorrow you become a four, what would you notice?" (a preferred-future question), or he can say, "What skills did you draw upon to get yourself to a three?" (a resource-talk question), or he can say, "When in your life were you the closest to ten on that scale? And what number were you then?" (a history-of-the-outcome question).

Again, a scale is a question that can go in any direction on a client's timeline. There are infinite ways to use scales, and they can assist you in becoming more inventive with your SFBT questions. We caution you, however, that if you do use scales to avoid the common pitfalls associated with them: interpreting the numbers, problem-solving, assessing, and using scales as a ladder.

Never Interpret Scaling Numbers

When having a scaling conversation, be careful not to make the assumption that you have an idea of what your client's desired outcome looks like when it's attached to a scale. For example, if a client named Ben says his desired outcome is happiness, which he currently experiences as a 5 out of 10 on a scale, don't assume that 5 means halfway to happiness for him.

While the meaning of a scale might seem mathematically obvious to you, it may not have the same meaning for your client.

Likewise, if Ben had told you he was an 8 out of 10 in regard to happiness, don't assume that 8 is a good enough number for him. On the flip side, if he said he was a 4 out of 10, don't assume that 4 isn't too difficult for him.

In essence, don't make any assumptions as to the meaning of a scaling number. Your clients are the ones who should attach the meaning, which we'll discuss later in this chapter.

Never Use Scales to Problem-Solve

Be careful not to ask a scaling question like, "How much pain are you in? On a scale of zero to ten, ten being the most pain and zero being the least pain, where are you on that scale?" This question utilizes the language associated with the problem (a.k.a., the pain), and places the emphasis on how bad the problem is (by putting the most pain at the top of the scale), and orients the client to think and consider the problem (the pain) as they answer this question.

In SFBT, we don't use scales as a problem-solving tool because we don't problem-solve at all.

Think of Laura, whom we've frequently used as an example in this book. There is nothing Elliott can do to solve the fact that Laura has a nonverbal son. The same can be said for clients with a terminal illness or those who have lost a loved one. If Elliott asked Laura a question like, "On a scale from one to ten, where ten is you're exactly the kind of mom you would like to be, that normal mom, and one is the exact opposite of that, where would you say you are now?" Now let's imagine that Laura replies with, "Um, I guess I would say I'm a three." This scaling question could quickly turn into a problem-solving tool (again, something we would never do) if the follow-up question became something like, "What do you think you could do that would help you move from a three to a four?" The emphasis on *doing* or what action is necessary to move up the scale automatically turns the focus of the question into problem-solving. Instead of focusing on what needs to be done, scaling questions should be used to highlight differences. A more appropriate follow-up question could be something like, "What would be the first thing you would notice that would let you know you had moved from a three to a four?" Or, "What difference would it make to you if you realized that somehow you had moved up the scale, even just a little bit, to a four?" These questions focus on the difference the movement would make rather than on the effort needed to make the movement.

Laura's problem isn't necessarily her nonverbal son; her problem is her broken heart associated with her nonverbal son. Sometimes people only associate broken hearts with the breakdown and difficulties of a romantic relationship, but broken hearts also occur with other significant disappointments in life. Your job is to heal those broken hearts. You're not a professional problem-solver, so a scale is not a problem-solving tool. You're a heart mender.

Never Use Scales to Assess

Similar to problem-solving, you don't want to use scales to assess your clients. Avoid questions like, "On a scale of zero to ten, how bad is your situation?"

Don't even use scales to assess clients positively: "On a scale of zero to ten, ten being you're as motivated as you can possibly be and zero being the exact opposite, where would you say you are today?" A "motivation scan" like that is still an assessment, and although it might seem positive, it still opens the door for negative assessments.

For example, if you had a client named Tiana and you told her, "I think you're very intelligent," you're letting her know that you're judging her intelligence, which ultimately comes across as an assessment, albeit a positive one.

Likewise, if you told Tiana, "I think you look great today," she would probably recognize that as a polite thing to say, and she might reply, "Thank you." But what if you didn't compliment her the next two times you saw her? It's not outside the bounds of reality that she might think, *Because my therapist didn't say anything, they don't think I look great today.*

Remember that once you start assessing people, the repercussions can turn negative very quickly, and you don't want that to happen. This is why we don't assess in SFBT, and scaling is no exception. You want to be very careful to only scale where the client sees themself in relation to their desired outcome. This initial question is the starting point to a conversation about difference or change. The differences or changes described should be related to noticing that the desired outcome is now a little more present. The scale isn't used to assess the presence of the desired outcome (something we can presuppose anyway), but instead it is used as a starting point for discussing signs of difference.

Never Use Scales as a Ladder

Be careful not to use scaling as a ladder, because ladders also lead to strategizing and problem-solving.

Let's say you have a client named Omar, and you ask him, "On a scale of zero to ten, ten being your desired outcome is present all of the time, and zero is it's never happening, where are you today?" (By the way, this is an appropriate way to ask a scale.)

"I'm at a two or three," Omar answers.

The scaling conversation becomes problematic if you then ask him something like, "So how can you move up from a two or three to a three or four?" That turns the scale into a ladder, which you're asking him to climb.

Remember that SFBT is a three-step process: desired outcome, description, and closing. Once you start asking questions about how to move up on a scale, you're no longer co-constructing a description; you're strategizing.

No psychotherapist has ever solved another person's problem. The only thing you can do is inspire and heal human hearts. If you use scales as a ladder, you're no longer talking to your clients' hearts. You're talking to their minds.

SFBT therapists are the most tempted to solve problems when working with scales. Resist that urge and remember the bounds of your job.

What If Clients Rig the Scale?

Some therapists get tripped up when their clients rig the scale. Don't let that faze you. Instead of arguing with their answer, keep the conversation going.

Let's say that during a follow-up session, you ask a client named Kristy, "On a scale from zero to ten, ten being your desired outcome is happening all the time and zero is the exact opposite, where are you at now?"

"I'm at a twenty!" Kristy exclaims.

Take her rigged answer and build on it. You could ask, "So what did you notice that let you know that life was staying at a twenty?" Or you could move Kristy's answer into the past and ask, "What have you done to get yourself to a twenty?"

Remember your clients' answers are always right. Use their language and stay grounded in your descriptions.

Using Scales across Descriptive Pathways

Let's examine a scaling conversation that Elliott had with Laura, whom you'll remember has a nonverbal son with a severe brain injury. To recap their previous desired-outcome discussion, Laura answered the best-hopes question by saying that she wanted her son to call her *Mom* (an impossible outcome). When then Elliott asked, "What difference would that make?" Laura established her desired outcome: to feel like a normal mom.

Elliott: If ten is you feeling like a normal mom all of the time, and zero is the exact opposite, where would you say you are today?

Laura: Probably a two.

Note that when Elliott asked this scaling question, he left zero undefined. Ten represents the desired outcome—in this case, feeling like a normal mom—and zero represents the opposite of that. Elliott left zero undefined because he's had no conversation with Laura about what zero looks like, and it doesn't matter that he hasn't. In SFBT, there's no reason to define zero.

Zero might be that Laura's in the corner crying every day, or zero might be that she's so hurt that she copes with alcohol or drugs. Zero could be a lot of different things, but you leave it at simply the opposite of ten. In order to define zero, you would have to ask your client several problem-solving questions, which you want to avoid.

When Laura told Elliott that she felt like a normal mom at a 2 out of 10 on a scale of her desired outcome being present, Elliott didn't panic or let himself think, *Oh, no! She's not very high on the scale!* The client's number is irrelevant. The only thing a scaling number does is gives you a fixed point with which to build questions.

Elliott is actually amazed by Laura for saying she's at a two. She has a son who was born with a difficult disability, and despite that she has figured out a way to muster the energy and strength to not only get out of bed but also get herself to a two.

In SFBT, you need to allow yourself to be easily amazed by people.

Elliott: Clearly, things aren't one hundred percent the way you'd like them to be. But since you said you were at a two, it also means that things aren't as bad as they could potentially be. What do you notice that lets yourself know that you might not be where you want to be today, but you're definitely not at a zero?

Laura: Well, my son is still alive, so I must be doing something right as a mom. And things are easier than how they were in the past.

Elliott: How do you know? What gives you a clue that they're easier?

Laura: I understand more about his brain injury, so that has made some things easier.

Elliott: What was your first clue that you were starting to gain an understanding about his brain injury?

Laura: Well, there was an occupational therapist who did a sensory assessment on him, and it clarified things I knew but didn't know how to explain. So I guess it validated me as a mom that I instinctively knew things about him and was doing what I needed to do. That was a pinnacle point for me.

Elliott: What difference did it make to you to have that validation as a mom?

Laura: It was a reminder that, even though so much of the care that's required for my son is not what a normal mom does, my "mom instinct" is still playing a really big role.

Elliott: And what difference does it make to you to know that, even though it's a different scenario, your mom instinct is still just as present and playing a big role as it would be in any other scenario?

Laura: It's made a big difference because, prior to that, I'd beaten myself up a lot about the fact that my maternal instinct wasn't working well, because I wasn't able to avoid my son getting the brain injury to begin with, so I felt like I'd let him down. So I guess it gave me a chance to look back and see that it wasn't true.

Elliott: What difference did that realization make to you?

Laura: I could finally let go of blaming myself, because actually my maternal instinct did do what it was supposed to do. So that was a big thing.

Did you notice how Elliott took the scale, and because he was genuinely amazed by Laura, he was able to ask questions that helped her articulate how arriving at a two happened? In this case, he took her scaling answer and went backward in her timeline, launching into a resource-talk description. Scales are very versatile in how they can be applied to the various description pathways.

Below, skipping to later in the session, notice how Elliott takes Laura's scaling answer and moves it forward in her timeline, shifting to a preferred-future description.

Elliott: So you're at a two now. If somehow you became a three, how would you notice it?

Laura: Maybe my thinking would be different.

Elliott: What would be different about your thinking?

Laura: I would be less focused on everything that sucks.

Elliott: What would you be more focused on instead?

Laura: All the parts that don't completely suck.

Elliott: Such as?

Laura: Maybe I'd be spending more time in the moment, like enjoying reading books to my son because he's very responsive in a delicious way. So maybe I'd be doing that and being smoochy rather than being on the Internet, googling things that get me down even more.

Elliott: And what difference would it make for you to be enjoying the moment, being smoochy, and in doing those sorts of things with your son? If you caught yourself doing those things more toward a three, what difference would that make to you?

Laura: I think I'd feel better, because who doesn't feel good when they're giving smooches? So I think it would just leave me with a bit of feeling good as I carried on with my day. Like, if I'm googling stuff and he's throwing up, it just kind of reinforces how much it all sucks. But if we're reading and he throws up, then I would be more like, "Oh, wee man, let's get you cleaned up," and maybe we'd go back to reading. So I guess the bits that I can't avoid wouldn't seem as impactful if I was doing those other in-the-moment things that I know my son and I both enjoy.

Notice how Elliott fought the urge to say, "How do you get to a three?" Instead, he treated Laura as if she already knew what a three looked like. And it turns out she did. When she described that three, it was magical. Nothing about her son changed, but everything about Laura did. She described reading to him and giving him smooches, even if they had a brief setback of him throwing up.

Laura's description didn't require any complimenting, pointing out, or encouragement on Elliott's part. It only required him to treat her like she could do what she wanted—feel like a normal mom.

Again, avoid the huge temptation to problem-solve with scales. Elliott would have been problem-solving by using a ladder if he'd said to Laura, "So you're at a two. What would it take for you to get to at least a three?" That becomes a "how-to" conversation.

Instead, Elliott said, "So you're at a two now. If somehow you became a three, how would you notice it?" Because he asked the scaling question that way, Laura was able to answer it by describing her desired outcome, rather than strategizing about how to arrive there.

Chapter 21

The Art of
Asking Questions

The Importance of
Mastering the Language

Elliott's catchphrase is, "You are always just one question away from making a difference." The reason that this idea is so important is because it highlights the fact that solution focused brief therapy is a questions-based model. That means to get good at it you have to master the art of asking questions—questions that produce change in your clients' lives, regardless of what brought them to therapy. Trust us, it's a hard skill to master, and we want to help you do just that.

Have you ever been stuck in a session because you couldn't think of the next question to ask? Perhaps your clients said something that threw you for a loop, and you didn't know how to respond. It's almost as if they went off script. Had they answered your question as planned, you would have known exactly what to say.

It's in those moments that you realize the theory doesn't help you. The technique doesn't help you. What you need is mastery of the language of psychotherapy. And that takes practice. It also takes knowing where you are in the session—which is why we created the diamond.

The best thing you can do to become fluent in the language of SFBT is to understand the process of the diamond and just ask the next question.

The beautiful thing is, once you become fluent, you can use this approach with any client, no matter their issue and no matter what they say that would otherwise throw you off course. When you're fluent in something, you don't get stuck in it. You just find a way to build another question and take another turn to talk.

Work hard to develop the fluency to come up with questions that, at any moment in the session, are connected to your clients' desired outcome and allow them to feel good about themselves. One helpful resource is a list of 101 questions in Appendix A.

The Client Who Didn't Drink on Tuesdays

Diving Deep with Elliott

In solution focused brief therapy, you ask questions so your clients can hear themselves say positive things about themselves—things that will make a difference in their world.

I once worked with a client who struggled with so much overdrinking that his belly was distended, and his skin had a yellowish hue. When I asked him the best-hopes question, he answered, "I need to be clean and sober." He'd made some bad decisions related to drinking, and he was in danger of losing his wife and family.

"When in your life are you the least likely to drink, or to drink less?" I asked.

"On Tuesdays," he said. "I tend to not drink as much or even at all on Tuesdays." When I asked him why, he explained, "I'm the assistant coach on my son's baseball team, and they have practice every Tuesday night, so I need to stay sober. That's also important because I drive my son to and from practice on Tuesdays."

"When did you realize that you were capable of making really good decisions once a week?" I asked.

He looked at me like I was crazy. "What do you mean?"

"Well, once a week, you make the decision to go to your son's baseball practice clean and sober, and you participate as any good and loving dad would. When did you realize you were capable of making good decisions once a week? That's pretty frequent."

He sat back in his chair, processing what I'd said. "I didn't think about it that way. I thought everybody would do the same thing I did."

"No, there are lots of stories in the news about people driving drunk while their kids were in the car. Also, people in your position might drink earlier in the day, thinking they could sleep it off in time, but you don't drink at all on Tuesdays."

He rubbed his jaw, thinking that over. "I guess that's true."

Once he realized that he could make good decisions once a week, it helped him make good decisions with more consistency. A year later he came back to my office and gave me his one-year sobriety chip. He thanked me, saying he was finally able to become sober when he learned to think about himself as being capable of making good decisions.

His sobriety chip remains one of my prized possessions.

Ask Questions That Make Your Client's Mood Escalate

Diving Deep with Elliott

If you want to make a difference in your clients' lives, you need to have a positive impact on what they see when they look at themselves. You need to ask questions that make them feel good when they answer them. Think about this in terms of creating a bit of a verbal hug.

Would you feel anything close to a verbal hug if someone asked you, "How did you get so fat?" Answering that would definitely not make you feel good, would it? But if someone asked you, "How did you get so handsome?" answering that *would* make you feel positive about yourself.

As I've mentioned before, I had a difficult relationship with my father, who was an aggressive and abusive man. Growing up, the one time I tried to go to therapy was when I was 18 years old. When my therapist asked what was wrong with me, right off the bat I felt horrible. Talking about what was wrong with me and how it felt to be punched in the face by my dad and how I struggled with anxiety and couldn't sleep and felt suicidal were the last things in the world that could have produced a positive feeling in me.

What if instead my therapist had asked, "How did you go through all of those difficult experiences and somehow find your way onto a college campus and become a college student?" Do you see how that question would have made me feel proud about myself? Do you see how it would have made me take credit for being good in this world?

In addition to creating questions that evoke positivity, hope, and excitement in your clients, each of your questions needs to be about the presence of the desired outcome. They should also be connected to the resources your clients have that can make that hoped-for future a reality.

For example, if you ask a client, "What are your best hopes from our talking?" and the client says, "I'd like to be happy," for the rest of the conversation, you need to ask questions that are more likely than not to produce an experience of happiness, as well as asking about the resources that can be utilized to do so.

Once you highlight your clients' talents, qualities, and skills, you're also reminding them that those resources have generalized applicability, meaning they can be applied unilaterally in their lives.

Remember Little Waco, who was the number one drug dealer in Waco, Texas, at the age of 14? He was able to stop dealing drugs because he learned that his true gift was being good at sales, and he used that gift to become a successful used-car salesman.

As an SFBT therapist, you need to be committed to asking your clients questions that make them feel good and proud of themselves—questions that they will grow from as they answer.

Keeping the diamond in mind, focus on just asking the next question in the process. Too often therapists try to ask the "right" question. Don't overthink it and get stuck in your head. Just ask the next question.

Honing the skill of building questions takes a lot of practice and effort, but if you want to make a positive impact on your clients' lives, you have to have a positive impact on the way they see themselves.

Don't Assess Your Clients or Ask Questions for Your Own Benefit

Solution focused questions are not designed to help you learn anything from your clients for your own benefit. This is a different mindset from how ordinary people ask questions. The number one reason people in the world ask questions is so they can gain something that will improve their lives.

If you like someone's shoes, you ask where you can buy them. If you enjoyed a home-cooked meal at your friend's house, you ask for the recipe. In SFBT, we don't do that. We don't ask questions for our own gain.

Let's say you have a friend named Julie. Instead of asking her, "Where did you buy that shirt?" you would ask, "When did you get so good at picking out really nice shirts?" Do you see how that question is for Julie's benefit and not your own? Do you see how it would help her feel positive and view herself in a different way?

It's like how Elliott asked his client who didn't drink on Tuesdays, "When did you realize that you were capable of making really good decisions once a week?" That question helped him see what he was doing well in life, despite his challenges.

Another reason clinicians ask questions is to do an assessment. In psychotherapy, an assessment question is asked to gauge the severity of the client's problem. For example, if you met with a client who had a drinking addiction, like Elliott's client, you'd start asking assessment questions like, "How often do you drink?" and "What are your triggers toward drinking?" and "How much alcohol do you consume when you drink?" and "How much money do you spend when you drink?"

In the clinical world, therapists are well trained at asking assessment questions. But when you're doing SFBT, you don't ask questions to assess because they don't produce a positive or difference-making impact on your clients, which is critical in this approach.

If you're not asking questions that change the way your clients view themselves, then you're not likely to make a difference in their lives. Learn to ask questions that allow them to re-experience themselves positively through their own answers.

Learn to Ask about the Smaller Details

A Closer Look with Adam

Some SFBT therapists tend to ask questions about big, broad topics. One of the most famous is, "What does that look like?" If you ask that big question, you're going to get a big answer. A typical response you might get to a big question like this is, "I don't know."

The reason clients might answer in this way is because the possible options to a question this big and open are endless. It's difficult for them to narrow their answer to just one small thing. It's simpler to just say, "I don't know," perhaps hoping that a more answerable question will follow. You can aid your clients in answering your questions by making your questions small and specific.

You need to learn to shrink the scope of what you're asking about. That's why Elliott and I ask, "What is the *very first* thing you would notice?" Asking about the first thing allows us to later ask, "What's the second thing you would notice?" and "What else would you notice?"

The smaller the details you can ask about, the more limits you can place on the topic, which allows you to break up big questions into smaller components. This expands your possibility of questions and prevents you from feeling like you're running out of conversation topics.

Another helpful tip is to think about the conversation like you would if it were a movie or still picture. Try to ask your clients questions that will help them visually set the scene.

For example, if you're co-constructing a description about your clients' preferred future, you can expand the conversation by asking, "Where would that happen?" and "Who else would be there?" and "What would the dialogue look like?" and "Would any pets be there?"

The more specific the questions you ask, the more your clients will be able to slowly unfold the scene that describes the presence of their best hopes.

Consider the small details asked about in the following example.

Therapist: What would be the very first thing you would notice on this day [that the desired outcome is present]?

Client: Well, I would wake up happy.

Therapist: What time would that be?

Client: Around seven o'clock.

Therapist: Would anyone else be present at seven o'clock when you wake up feeling happy?

Client: Yeah, my partner would be lying next to me.

Therapist: Would they be awake or asleep? Are they a morning bird or night owl?

The smaller you can make your questions, the more details and scene-setting your clients will be able to describe. Remember, this is a change-focused approach. With each detail that your clients articulate, they are connecting that detail to the presence of their desired outcome. In some sense, they are broadening their neural pathways to include more and more details that are connected to exactly what they want.

Because each of the very small details are meaningfully connected to the desired outcome, your clients are more likely to notice them as they leave the session to go about living their everyday lives. And the more your clients notice these details, the more likely they are to remember that they are connected to their desired outcome.

They will begin to see the small details differently, they will have confirmation that the desired outcome is present in their lives, and they will begin behaving differently as a result of noticing these small but meaningful changes. The change that your clients achieved linguistically during the session will also manifest outside the session right before their eyes.

The Most Powerful Word in the SFBT Vocabulary

Diving Deep with Elliott

I recently saw a young woman who was struggling with intense levels of fear that were holding her back from making significant decisions and taking important actions in her life.

When I asked her what she hoped to achieve from being in therapy, she said, "I don't even know. I'm depressed. I'm anxious. I'm fearful. And I don't want to alarm you, but I've had thoughts about ending my life. I'm not at *risk* of ending my life," she clarified. "I just don't care about it anymore because I don't know how to get rid of this fear."

How did I handle this situation? I asked the most powerful question in solution focused brief therapy. In fact, this question holds the most powerful *word* in SFBT. I asked, "What would you like to feel instead?"

People focus so much on problems that it's hard for them to answer questions related to what they'd like to achieve unless they're put in the context of what they'd like to achieve *instead* of their problems.

When I first asked this young woman what she'd like to achieve, she couldn't give me a direct answer. She just started rattling off all the details of her problem and the symptoms connected to it, which were really significant.

But the real therapy didn't begin for her—the process of change didn't start happening—until I asked, "What would you like to feel *instead*? If somehow all of those problems went away, what would you like to have in their place?"

"I don't know," she replied.

"So what do you think?" I prodded gently.

"I'd like to be confident," she finally answered. "I'd like to be strong. And I'd like to be the best me that I can be."

Now she was giving me language I could use to ask her about the preferred future, which I did: "Suppose you woke up tomorrow and you were confident and strong and the best version of you that you could be. What's the first thing you would notice?"

We went about doing a description, which couldn't have happened unless I had first asked, "What would you like to feel *instead*?"

When a therapist asks the best-hopes question and the client replies by talking about problems, the therapist has the misconception that the client can't establish the desired outcome without talking about problems first, when actually what the client needs is for the therapist to ask, "What would you like to feel/be/do *instead*?"

By the end of our session, the young woman was very pleased with the conversation we'd just had. "Is it normal that I already feel better?" she said.

A few hours later, she sent me a really nice e-mail explaining how I'd helped to shift her focus from what was bothering her to what she wanted to achieve. "I'd never thought about it in that way before," she said. She closed the e-mail by saying she was already looking forward to our next conversation.

As you begin each session, don't get sucked into the trap of thinking your clients can't answer your best-hopes question because they need to talk about their problems first. This is a time for you to reach into your solution focused language and pull out a question that contains the most powerful word in SFBT: *instead*. Ask your clients what they would like to be experiencing *instead* and watch the magic unfold.

Don't Worry about
Silence or Disparaging Answers

Even clients who refuse to talk or talk very little are doing the work of SFBT; they're just answering your questions in their head.

Let's say you asked, "How did you learn to do that?" Your clients can't help but try to figure out the reason, and meanwhile their mood escalates because SFBT questions make people feel good about themselves.

When your clients say their answers aloud, that might help you, but it actually makes no difference to them because they have thought through their answers anyway, which still triggers the change-making process.

On a similar note, don't get discouraged if your clients' answers are sometimes negative or overly self-critical. What they say is often different from what they are thinking. Before speaking aloud, they put their answer through the filter of "But can I tell this person this?" or "How do I actually say this?" As a result, you sometimes have no idea what their real answer is, but rest assured that your clients are still building a transformative narrative internally.

You're only getting the tip of the iceberg with what your clients say, and you might not see the full payoff of how SFBT is helping them during the session. But you can count on the fact that the work of transformation is continuing to happen as they leave your office and engage in the real world.

Have faith in the process, maintain a strong belief in your clients, and trust in their capability to achieve their best hopes.

Argue without Offending

Diving Deep with Elliott

In solution focused work, you need to master the art of confronting your clients' reality without offending them.

I was once conducting a training where a therapist told me about a client that she was at a loss with. After she'd co-constructed a preferred-future description with him, in which he talked about being a good father, he said, "Well, I'm sure Hitler went home and was a great dad. So if I go home and am a great dad, that doesn't mean I'm not a jerk."

This therapist wanted my advice on how I would have handled this situation or ones like it where clients make extremely negative self-comparisons.

Now, first off, Adolf Hitler never raised any children, but that's beside the point. It's not the kind of reality I recommend arguing about with your clients. What you need to do is dispute the reality of how they view themselves.

If I'd been in this therapist's shoes and my client had just compared himself with Hitler, I'd be thinking, *I cannot allow this man to ever again use his own name and Hitler in the same sentence.* To distance him from that comparison, I'd start asking questions that got to the root of "But how are you different?"

I would have said something like, "You're right. Hitler probably was very good to the people around him behind closed doors and a murderous jerk everywhere else. So let's imagine you're just the same. You're kind behind closed doors and a bit of a rage monster in public. But let's say this miracle changes that, and all of a sudden your ability to be good only behind closed doors failed, and it started seeping into other areas of your life. What would you notice that would tell you that your goodness wasn't restricted to interactions with your children? How would you notice that it wasn't containable and that it leaked out?"

With those questions, I would have removed this man's ability to compare himself to Hitler any longer. I'd have challenged his reality that everyone can do good things behind closed doors and be jerks in public. And I would have challenged that reality without offending him.

Always try to separate your clients from their ability to make negative self-comparisons. Help them recognize that change is possible and goodness can grow. If they believe they're bad, they're more likely to behave as bad. But when they believe they're good, they're much more likely to behave as good.

How to Ask
Sensitive and Difficult Questions

Diving Deep with Elliott

A therapist once asked me how solution focused brief therapy could help homeless people. He said, "It seems strange to ask, 'What will it look like when you aren't homeless?'"

I agreed with him. Not only would that seem strange, but it would also be hurtful.

First of all, I wouldn't ask that question. I actually have a lot of experience working with homeless people; I volunteered at a homeless center for several years in my practice. Many of our conversations went like this:

"What are your best hopes from our talking?"

"I don't want to be homeless anymore."

"What would you rather be?"

"I'd rather live in a big old mansion."

"What difference would it make for you to be living in a big old mansion?"

"Well, I'd be happy. I would have peace, joy, and security."

I would then ask a really hard question: "Let's suppose you woke up tomorrow and you were on your way to living a life with happiness, peace, joy, and security, but it didn't wait for you to have a home. It started happening in your life now. What's the first thing you would notice?"

That would be my way of honoring that these homeless people are in a really difficult situation while also doing my job to come up with a question to help them transform that really difficult situation.

For the record, one of the ways Insoo Kim Berg demonstrated the effectiveness of SFBT was by going to a section of Milwaukee, Wisconsin, and asking the homeless community solution focused questions. They got sober quicker and stayed sober longer than they had with AA.

Afterword

Thank you for investing your time and energy into reading this book. We hope you have found new insights and understanding that will help you to help your clients achieve meaningful outcomes in their lives. Although we have studied and researched extensively for over a decade to develop the ideas in this book, we understand that it is really our clients who teach us how to do this approach well. Therefore, we hope you will take these ideas into your work, and we hope that you will never forget to be guided by the language of your clients.

We also feel compelled to state that we believe that solution focused brief therapy is always evolving—change is constant, after all. We feel honored to stand on the shoulders of giants such as Steve de Shazer, Insoo Kim Berg, Yvonne Dolan, and Eve Lipchik. There is no way we could have written this book or developed these ideas without their groundbreaking work! In addition, we are indebted to Chris Iveson, Evan George, and Harvey Ratner (The Brief Boys) for pushing us another step forward. Their ability to evolve the approach gave us permission to entertain our own ideas and to grow in confidence to share those ideas with the world. We hope that you, as the reader, have learned something from our current evolution, but we hope you have felt the stirrings of new questions and new ideas of your own. We hope you will let those ideas grow and develop and that in 5, 10, or 15 years we will be reading your book and learning from your thoughts and research. We hope this book gives you permission to push SFBT to the next level. We hope this book is only one step to helping more and more people move toward their desired outcomes!

We also hope the diamond model can serve as a unifying language for solution focused practitioners. Whether you are new and learning this approach for the first time, or if you are a well-seasoned practitioner who has been practicing SFBT for decades, we hope this book has brought clarity to how you can work with clients to achieve lasting change. We hope you design research studies, prepare workshops and trainings, and conduct therapy using the principles from the diamond model. We have found this approach to radically change people's lives and we hope that your life has been changed, for the better, because of this book.

Beyond just the writings about SFBT, we hope our relationship and friendship have had a positive impact on you. It is hard to write so personally, but in a world that is filled with divisiveness, we feel compelled to show that difference doesn't need to breed contempt. Working with each other has been one of the greatest blessings we have each enjoyed. Only as we have respected and cherished our differences have we truly been able to reach our full potential. We hope you view differences between you and your clients as opportunities to be amazed. We hope you view differences between you and your colleagues as opportunities to be taught. We hope you are blessed with amazing growth as you embrace, rather than fear, difference! We hope each of you will ADOPT the diamond stance and make the world better by celebrating each person's unique contribution!

Finally, we hope you will each stay in touch and be a part of our growing community. The Solution Focused Universe (SFU) is the home of the SFBT diamond model. This community is a place of ongoing learning and engagement. The SFU is the largest solution focused community in the world and creates innovative training material each month. The SFU has members from all livable continents. Clinicians who previously felt isolated and alone in their solution focused journey now have a thriving community to draw strength and support from. We hope we get to see you there and learn from and with you.

Thank you again for letting us be a part of your solution focused journey through this book. We wish you all the best in all your solution focused pursuits.

Appendix A

Elliott Connie's 101
Solution Focused Questions

Desired-Outcome Questions

1. What are your best hopes from our work together?
2. What difference would you like this session to make for you?
3. What would the person who suggested you come here hope to be different for you as a result of us meeting?
4. What would your closest friend hope to be different for you as a result of us meeting?
5. What differences would you hope would happen in your life as a result of us talking?
6. What do you wish would be different as a result of you being here?
7. What do you think? (This is often asked in response to clients who say, "I don't know.")
8. If you did know, then what?
9. If I asked the person in your life who knows you best, what do you think they'd say?
10. What do you imagine?
11. If I had asked you this question when you did know, what would you have said?
12. What would you have said if I asked you this question on the day you first called me to schedule this appointment?
13. If I had asked you that question when you were at your most hopeful and motivated, what would you have said?
14. What would you like instead?

Resource-Talk Questions

15. What do you do for fun?
16. What do you do for a living?
17. How did you become good at that?
18. What did it take to be good at that?
19. What has it taken to stay good at that?
20. What would the closest person to you say is their favorite thing about you?
21. How do you show the people in your life that you care about them?
22. What are you most proud of about yourself?
23. What would the people who raised you say they are most proud of about the adult you have become?
24. What has improved since you scheduled this appointment?
25. How did you do that?
26. What did you draw upon to help that thing improve?
27. When did you first notice that things were improving?
28. Were you surprised to see these things improving?
29. Who in your life was not surprised to see this improving?
30. What do you know about yourself that lets you know you can achieve what you want?
31. What do you know about the problem that lets you know it can be solved? And that you can solve it?

Resource Talk with Couples

32. How did you meet?
33. Once you met, how did you first notice the potential for a long-term relationship?
34. How did you know that your partner was also interested?
35. What did you first do to let your partner know you were interested?
36. What did you notice your partner doing that let you know they enjoyed the early days of this relationship?
37. How did you let them know you were pleased about their enjoyment?
38. When did you each first notice that this relationship had a future?
39. What is your favorite thing about your partner?
40. What are you most proud of about the relationship you have created?

41. What are you most pleased that your children get to see about your relationship?

42. What did each of you do to grow the relationship from when you first met to the happiest times?

43. How did you maintain those happy times before the problem started?

44. Once the problem started, what did each of you do to help solve it?

45. What made you try to solve the problem instead of giving up on the relationship?

46. What makes you think trying, and not giving up, is a good thing?

Coping with the Problem/
When the Client Talks about the Problem

47. What would you like to experience instead of the problem?

48. How have you dealt with the problem while it has been present?

49. When has the problem diminished or become less intense?

50. What role did you play in the problem diminishing or going away?

51. What was different about you while the problem was gone or less intense?

52. Who else noticed that the problem was going away or becoming less intense?

53. When did you first notice the problem was going away or diminishing?

54. How did they notice the problem had gone away or become less intense?

55. What difference did the problem going away or becoming less intense make in that person's life?

56. What difference did that person noticing the problem going away make for you?

Preferred-Future Description Questions

57. Suppose you went to sleep one night and a miracle happened that solved all of the problems that led you into my office. What is the first thing you would notice?

58. If you woke up tomorrow and your best hopes had become a reality, what would you first notice?

59. If the changes that you noticed, even before the session, continued, what would you notice?

60. If the problem kept diminishing and even went away, and your best hopes replaced it, what would you notice?
61. If those differences you, and those close to you, noticed once the problem went away were to continue, what would you notice?
62. What time would it be?
63. What else?
64. What would you do next?
65. What would you notice next?
66. Would you consider this a good thing?
67. What difference would that make?
68. Would that please you?
69. How would you show that you were pleased to those close to you?
70. How would those close to you notice you were pleased?
71. How would those close to you let you know their life had improved as well?
72. If your lost loved one were looking down, what would they notice that would make them pleased?

Scaling Questions

73. On a scale of zero to ten, with ten representing your desired outcome has been realized and zero is the opposite, where are you today?
74. On a scale of one to ten, where ten represents your desired outcome being completely realized and one is the problem at its worst, where are you today?
75. What puts you at that number?
76. How do you know you're not at zero?
77. What have you done to prevent the situation from going down on the scale?
78. If you moved one point on the scale toward the realization of your desired outcome, what is the first thing you would notice?
79. If you moved up on the scale slightly, what would you notice?
80. What have you done to get yourself to the number you are currently at?
81. What else have you done to get yourself to that number?
82. Who has noticed you progressing up the scale?
83. What difference has it made to those close to you to see you progress?

84. What difference would it make to those close to you for you to continue this progress?

85. What other differences would it make to them for you to continue up the scale?

86. What would you notice as clues that you were progressing?

87. How would you show you were progressing?

88. How would you demonstrate that you were pleased to be progressing?

89. How would those close to you notice you were pleased to be progressing?

90. How would they notice you had noticed your positive impact on them?

Follow-Up Session Questions

91. What's been better since our last session?

92. How'd you do that?

93. How did you hold on to enough hope for change and come back to therapy, even though things got worse?

94. What skills did you draw upon to make those changes since our last session?

95. What areas of your life got better other than the one we discussed in our last session?

96. What's been better since we last met?

97. What role did you play in things getting better since we last met?

98. What role did others play?

99. What are your best hopes for this session?

100. What does that progress do to your thoughts about the future?

101. Was this change a big surprise or a little surprise?

Appendix B

Transcript of Elliott's Session with Liz

Annotations by Adam

Because SFBT happens at the language level, and because it is through language that clients change, we want to demonstrate how change happens by using an actual SFBT session. There is no better way to learn the language of SFBT than to study it. For this reason we have included an entire SFBT session below. This one was conducted virtually, and we have supplemented this session dialogue with commentary about what might be going on in the head of an SFBT therapist, how decisions are made about what language to use and what language to leave behind. We hope that this commentary will help you gain fluency as you get a behind-the-scenes look at how SFBT co-construction is formulated.

By way of functionality, we added numbers next to each of the therapist's and client's utterances. These numbers are used as reference points in the commentary throughout the document to orient the reader to specific language mentioned in the description.

For confidentiality reasons, the client's name has been changed.

001	Elliott	So what are your best hopes from our chat today?

This is always the way that we start sessions. We have found this to be an effective way to begin a conversation that will lead to identifying the client's desired outcome, or desired transformation.

002	Liz	Become a nonsmoker, today.

It would be easy to panic at this point. Liz just mentioned something that Elliott doesn't have much control over; he can't make Liz stop smoking. However, Liz has begun to identify a transformation she would like to make. It will be important for Elliott to use this language in his next question in order to continue to co-construct a new reality. Remember, this approach is a change-oriented approach.

003	Elliott	To become a nonsmoker today. And if you became a nonsmoker today, what difference would it make in your life?

Notice that Elliott takes Liz completely seriously. If you say something like, "Maybe we should talk about something a little more realistic" or "Well, maybe that can't happen today, but at some point . . ." then you inadvertently argue with your clients about what they want. This work isn't about challenging your clients; rather it is about working WITH them.

Elliott takes Liz's answer and asks about the difference it would make. By asking about difference, he is getting closer to really understanding the transformation she would like in her life. Stopping smoking is a change but not a transformation. A transformation is the WHY that Liz is hoping to achieve by using the strategy of stopping smoking.

004	Liz	Oh, I would feel free of this addiction.
005	Elliott	You'd feel free of this addiction?

This is a clarifying question. Even in these questions, you want to make sure to use as much of the client's language as possible.

006	Liz	Yes.
007	Elliott	And what would be different about you as you felt free?

Again, Elliott is asking about difference. It is worthwhile to notice how many times the word different *is used in a session. Because this is a change-oriented approach, you need to be consistently asking about the change (transformation) the client wants.*

Elliott is basically asking Liz the same question he asked in utterance 005. However, it is now a very different question because it involves the word free. *He is now talking to the version of Liz that is able to envision herself as free from addiction.*

008   Liz   What would be different about me? I always have trouble with these questions.

009   Elliott   That's why I ask them.

This is a very Elliott response! You have to be completely yourself in these sessions, and Elliott is so good at doing that.

010   Liz   Yeah. Right. What would be different? I would feel more that I was out of its control. I would be gaining back some of my own power.

011   Elliott   You'd be gaining back some of your own power?

Again, this is another clarifying question. This serves to provide confirmation that Elliott and Liz are grounding on the same points and that they are co-constructing in a way that is right for the client. Inserting these confirmation questions into the session helps to prevent the therapist from inserting things that aren't approved by the client. These questions really show the question-by-question development of the conversation.

012   Liz   Yes.

013   Elliott   Okay. And, Liz, when in your life do you remember having—you said, "gaining back"—the most of your own power?

This is a beautiful question! This question highlights that whenever your clients say they would like to have something (whenever they voice their desired outcome/transformation), you have to believe that they have at least had a small portion of that desired outcome at some point in their life. You can hear in this question a presupposition that Liz has had power before. Even though she mentioned "gaining back some of my own power," this question could still have been asked with the same presupposition embedded. This is the type of confidence we want to have in our clients when we are working from this perspective.

014   Liz   I'm going to say back when I was as young as five or six.

015   Elliott   As young as five or six. And if I had known you, when you were around five or six, what would I have seen that would have told me this is a person with a sense of power and control?

Elliott begins this utterance with a formulation, or summary, of what Liz just said. Again, this serves a grounding purpose and ensures they are on the same page. He then moves on to a presuppositional question that assumes he would have been able to notice something that told him Liz had power and control.

This question shows how well Elliott holds on to information. Liz mentioned in utterance 010 that she would like to be out of addiction's control. Elliott used the word control *from that utterance even though they had only been using the word* power *since that time. The more you can remember and use the specific words from your client, even many utterances later, the more closely you are sticking to the description they want to develop.*

016   Liz   What would you have seen? I was very . . . I was much looser than I am now. I was very direct. I'm still direct. Wait a minute, I wasn't as . . . I was going to say inhibited. Yep. Okay. I wasn't inhibited. I was just more centered.

017   Elliott   Ah, you're just more centered. Okay. So if a miracle happened that somehow reawakened that five- or six-year-old version of yourself inside of you—and you got to keep all the memories and experiences you've gotten along the way—and that part that has power and is in control just comes back, just like that [*snaps fingers*]. When you woke up the next day, what's the first thing you'd notice that let you know you were back to being this version of yourself?

Many people will recognize this question as a version of the miracle question. Please don't read this question as a technique. Elliott could not have asked this question to anyone besides Liz. He was very masterful at incorporating many of Liz's words into this very specific question. Five- or six-year-old version, power, and control *were all used because Liz had taught Elliott what her desired transformation was. This question is only because it is about exactly what Liz wants.*

It is also important to note that we don't really talk about this kind of question as a miracle question. Although it is a miracle question, we prefer to talk about this question as one version of a future-of-the-outcome (preferred-future) question. This question is asking Liz to consider what life would be like in the future when her desired transformation is present. Elliott could have easily transitioned to the future by asking a different question. The important thing is that Elliott uses Liz's language and begins the sequence of getting a detailed description of her desired outcome.

018   Liz   [*With a smile on her face*] Happy.

019   Elliott   Okay. What time would it be that you'd wake up happy?

This question gets to a very specific level of detail. The more detailed you can be, the better.

Also, you can see that even in a very simple question, Elliott is careful to include Liz's language. Not just any of her language, the language that is consistent with the presence of her desired outcome.

020   Liz   What time in the morning?

021   Elliott   Yeah.

022   Liz   Five, six.

023   Elliott   Closer to five, closer to six, on a day when you wake up happy, what do you think?

Again, even when the question is really simple, Elliott is careful to use the desired-outcome language. He also won't co-construct something without Liz giving specific permission through her language.

024   Liz   Six.

025   Elliott   Six. And when you woke up at six o'clock, what's the very first clue you might get that would let you know you were happy?

This question includes something really important. The important word here is first. *When you add these superlative words (e.g., first, most, best, etc.), you orient the client to something very specific. These words help to make the question more answerable. In contrast, often clinicians will ask things like, "When you wake up happy, what would that look like?" A question like this is too general and very difficult to answer; the response could really include anything. When you say, "What is the first thing you would notice," you orient the client to think of and articulate one specific thing. These specific responses also serve the larger function of contributing to the very detailed description being developed.*

Also, note the "happy" language is still used directly. The more we can infuse the language, the better.

026	Liz	I'd be smiling.
027	Elliott	Okay. And after you caught this smile—is there anybody around at this time at, at six o'clock?

It is interesting to see Elliott interrupt his own question here. He was asking a question that included "smiling," then interrupted to ask a different question.

This is what we refer to as a scene-setting question. "Is there anybody around at six o'clock?" helps Elliott know if he should include anyone else's perspective in the description. Some might feel self-conscious about the "no" response to this question. As you will see in the next question, Elliott doesn't worry about it, but just returns to the previously half-formed question. We often emphasize the importance of being genuine. Elliott wanted to know if anyone else was around, and it would be disingenuous not to ask.

026	Liz	No.
029	Elliott	No, just you. So after you caught this smile, what's the first thing you might do?

Again, notice the superlative first.

030	Liz	Get up and go to the bathroom.
031	Elliott	Normal thing to do first thing in the morning. And after you came out of the bathroom, what would be something you might do that would just fit for someone who had power and control and was centered in all the ways that were right for them?

You can see here that Elliott just acknowledges something that could have been awkward, but he normalizes the response. He then quickly moves past the bathroom and back to the desired outcome. He is purposeful to allow private things to be private. He is equally purposeful about reintroducing the language of the desired outcome back into the session. This helps reorient the client back to the co-constructed conversation that is happening.

Again, notice the "just fit" language. This serves to narrow the focus of the client to the small details. Elliott continues to use the words power, control, *and* centered. *Over and over.*

032   Liz   I'd be dancing across the room.

033   Elliott   Would you really?

034   Liz   Yes.

035   Elliott   Do you enjoy dancing?

This is a very simple question, but it is an important scene-setting question. If Liz enjoys dancing, Elliott will know that he should keep this language in the session. If the answer is no, he should move on to other more important things. These simple questions are great ways to learn the language of clients.

036   Liz   Haven't done it in a hundred years, but I used to, yes.

I just want to point out that this answer is evidence that Liz is answering the questions as the five- or six-year-old version of herself. Her answer, dancing, was something that she used to do, not something that she has a regular practice of doing. Statements like this can often be overlooked, but they should be appreciated for the significance of their meaning.

037   Elliott   You used to. And what would be the type of, like— just before you started dancing, how would you know that this is the type of morning where you're about to be dancing?

You can see that Elliott again begins this utterance with a formulation that preserves Liz's language exactly. He then asks a question after interrupting his partially constructed question. Elliott is really good at self-regulating in the moment and changing his questions. This is a very difficult skill that is hard to do in real time.

There is a presupposition in the question, one that assumes Liz will know that this is a morning when she is just about to dance. You can see from the response below that Liz doesn't question the presupposition but instead works to answer the question that presupposes change, a change that is consistent with the powerful, in-control version of herself.

038   Liz   How would I know? I don't know. I just do it. I don't know. I just do it. I don't, uh, ha! Okay, I haven't paid attention to that. I just do it.

| 039 | Elliott | Well, now that you are paying attention to it, what do you think would be the clue that would let you know that this is a morning where you're about to dance in a way that you haven't in one hundred years? |

Did you notice that Liz has predominantly been using present tense language in her answers? She broke that trend in utterance 038 by noticing the process and commenting briefly about the process, "Uh, ha! I haven't paid attention to that." At this point, Elliott also switches his language to present tense language to say, "Now that you are paying attention to it . . . " He also brings back her language from utterance 036 about not dancing for 100 years.

| 040 | Liz | [*Long pause.*] I would feel light. My body would feel light. My inner self would feel free and light. |
| 041 | Elliott | Right, right. And would you be pleased by this? |

Again, you can see the grounding happening here. Elliott continually checks in to make sure they are building a conversation that is right for Liz.

| 042 | Liz | Yes. |
| 043 | Elliott | You would! And as you took this lightness and this inner self and sprang into this dance, what difference would it make for you to catch yourself dancing across the room? |

Even though Elliott uses the word difference *here again, this* difference *serves a different function. Previously (see utterance 007) Elliott used the word* different, *but he was asking about what would be different about Liz. In this instance, Elliott is asking a meaning-making question. He is asking Liz to consider the impact or significance that dancing would have. We should never leave SFBT sessions without asking the client at some point to make meaning of the conversation and details that are being described. This takes the conversation about difference and makes it make a difference.*

044	Liz	What difference would it make? I'd just be ecstatic.
045	Elliott	You would?
046	Liz	I would.
047	Elliott	How would you know you were dancing with this ecstatic feeling?

This may seem like a redundant question, but again, the more details you can help the client articulate, the more likely they are to see these signs in their everyday life. This kind of conversation is viewed as a dry rehearsal for their actual life in the presence of their desired outcome.

On another note, SFBT is often critiqued by some who claim it doesn't focus on or allow clients to talk about their feelings/ emotions. This is untrue! Clients can talk about anything they would like to talk about. We often say that every answer given by the client is exactly the right answer. Elliott is using feeling language, because this is the exact right thing to ask about since the client brought it up.

048   Liz   By how I'm feeling and what I'm doing.

049   Elliott   Okay. And how would you be able to describe that feeling as it was happening right then?

It is important to notice that, although Liz gave an answer, more clarification is needed. Her answer was vague and non-descript. A good SFBT therapist will ask for more clarity in situations like this, just like Elliott does.

050   Liz   [*Long pause.*] Perfect peace.

051   Elliott   Perfect peace. And how would you know that was perfect peace? You haven't had it— [*Liz laughs a little.*] How would, how would you know, what would be a clue to you that, as you were dancing, you had perfect peace?

You can tell that Elliott began mentioning that Liz hadn't had perfect peace in a long time. However, she didn't mention this before. She did mention that she hadn't had power or control like this since she was five or six years old. She did mention that she hadn't danced in 100 years. But she didn't mention she hadn't had peace. Therefore, it is good that Elliott interrupted himself and changed the way he was asking this question. I would argue that good therapists feel okay changing direction, even in midsentence.

052   Liz   I can describe it; I can't come up with one word for it.

053   Elliott   Sure, no. Of course.

054   Liz   I wouldn't care what anybody else—there's nobody else there, but I wouldn't be caring if there was.

055   Elliott   You wouldn't care at all, would you?

Another really well-used formulation that solidifies and grounds the detail that, when Liz has power and control, she doesn't care about what other people think.

056   Liz   No, I wouldn't.

057	Elliott	And now [*Elliott makes a slight dance move*]—
058	Liz	[*Liz talking over Elliott*] That's certainly one.
059	Elliott	Right? What else?

Liz's response of "That's certainly one" implies that this is only one sign that would let her know she was experiencing perfect peace. This allows Elliott to automatically ask about the other signs of perfect peace with the "What else?" question. This is a very common SFBT question. Again, the more details, the better. However, in this case, Liz really left the door wide open!

| 060 | Liz | What else? I shouldn't have said that, "That's certainly one." |
| 061 | Elliott | Not to me! I'm the wrong person to say that to, ma'am. |

You can really see Elliott's personality coming through here. SFBT should be a genuine conversation with a genuine therapist. If you use humor in everyday life, like Elliott does, you shouldn't leave it out of the room. Authenticity is vital in this work.

062	Liz	I'm getting that pretty quick. [*Both Elliott and Liz laugh.*] Oh, what else? Is it okay if I take a minute to think?
063	Elliott	It's more than okay to take a minute to think.
064	Liz	Oh, okay. [*Long pause.*] I would be feeling that I really, really want to be doing that. Just that, that bubbling thing while I'm doing it. Yeah.
065	Elliott	Just right then in that moment?
066	Liz	Yep.
067	Elliott	Okay. And how long would this dancing bit last?
068	Liz	Probably until I tired out at the other side of the room. [*Elliott laughs.*] I only stretched the hundred years by about twenty-five. So . . .
069	Elliott	Yes, ma'am. And after the dancing bit ended, you're all the way on the other side of the room, and you realize like, *I didn't care at all who was in the room with me, if anybody were watching. I'm centered and I have this peace, and I'm ecstatic.* What's the very next thing you might catch yourself doing?

Notice that the desired-outcome words are still being repeated, even at utterance 069. Centered, peace, *and* ecstatic *are still the focus of the session. Often when clients give these kind of details, SFBT therapists may take the bait and ask many follow-up questions about these details. They may be tempted to ask, "What difference would it make to be dancing in this way?" or something like that. Although this is an SFBT question, it doesn't really build the desired-outcome description. There is real discipline required to stay focused on the description of the desired outcome. This is often where the masters of SFBT are separated from the beginners.*

070	Liz	Having a coffee. And I have to be honest, I thought, having a coffee and a cigarette.

Do you see that change is already happening? We believe that language creates reality. She has been talking about herself as a nonsmoker in the version of powerful, in control, and ecstatic. At this moment, she realized that the old answer was incompatible with this version of herself. She is already becoming a different version of herself.

071	Elliott	But you said having a coffee. So on your way to the coffee, how would you know that you were heading to the coffee in a way that was just right for this version of yourself that was light and ecstatic and no longer cared what other people said?

This is one of my favorite responses in this session. Elliott simply says, "But you said having a coffee." Do you see that Elliott does not get pulled into a conversation about why she wanted to say cigarette too? Do you see that he doesn't have to "argue" with Liz about how she is different now, or that this answer no longer applies? He simply acknowledges the language she DID use. He then returns to his job by asking another question about the desired-outcome description.

072	Liz	So I guess I would just be almost floating out there, not really worried about what dust is there or whatever.
073	Elliott	Right. You'd be doing this floating thing and not noticing like dust and stuff like that, you said?

This is another question that seeks to ensure that Elliott understood what Liz had said. Because this session was conducted virtually, it may have been a little difficult for Elliott to hear and understand everything. It is always better to clarify than to assume.

074 Liz   Yeah.

075 Elliott   Okay.

076 Liz   Housework type stuff.

077 Elliott   Yes, ma'am. And throughout the course of your life, who would you say is the person that has known you the absolute best?

This is another scene-setting question. One of the powerful effects of SFBT is that clients get to describe the difference their desired outcome would have on the people around them. Important people are contributors to conversations.

078 Liz   My husband.

079 Elliott   Your husband—his name, please?

080 Liz   Bill.

081 Elliott   Bill. And is Bill still around?

This is another example of Elliott's confidence. This could be a difficult question for many people to ask. But because Elliott sees his job as getting details, he will often need to ask difficult questions in order to get answers.

082 Liz   No. He died.

083 Elliott   When did he die?

This simple but challenging question gives Elliott a lot of information about how to include Bill in the conversation. He knows that he needs Bill's perspective to be a hypothetical perspective, since he is not able to see the actions Liz is taking. He knows Bill's perspective is one that is accurate, since Liz mentioned that he knew her best. We can't shy away from difficult questions if we need the answers to do our jobs well.

084 Liz   2005.

085 Elliott   2005. Okay, okay. So if Bill were watching you make this floating move from wherever you finished dancing toward the coffee, what would be a clue to him that you were at your very, very best doing this floating thing toward the coffee?

This is a masterful question! Elliott reimmerses Liz into the description after the short detour about Bill. Elliott remembers the tiniest detail, like the fact that Liz didn't know where she would finish dancing, but it would just end when she got tired. He incorporated this previous unknown location into the question. He also remembered that Liz hadn't even made it to the coffee yet; she was simply moving toward the coffee. He doesn't forget or change any of the details of the description. This is Liz's description, and it should stay that way.

There is also a presupposition that Bill would notice. Elliott doesn't ask, "Would Bill notice?" He assumes that, because Bill knew her the best, he would notice a difference in Liz. Holding this view that important people will notice change is one of the foundations that SFBT is built on.

086	Liz	Well, just knowing he's never seen me do it before.
087	Elliott	Hmm, so how would he know if he's never seen you do it? He knows you really well, though. How would he know that you were doing this thing that really fit well for you?

It is really interesting that Elliott switched to present tense here. Liz also spoke in present tense in utterance 086. It is interesting because they are talking about someone who has already passed away as though he were there at this moment. This change in tense is common in SFBT sessions when people are really putting themselves into the situation being described. I would suggest that this is a sign of change.

088	Liz	How would he know?
089	Elliott	Yeah.
090	Liz	My whole demeanor. The look on my face would be different. Everything.
091	Elliott	Right, right. And what's the type of look that Bill would recognize, *That's my wife when she's just at her best*?

I don't think there is anything that can be said about this question except can you imagine describing what your husband, the person who knows you the best, would say about you at your very best? This is way bigger than floating. This is way bigger than coffee. This is Liz at her very best! Elliott often talks about how the purpose of SFBT is to inspire people. It is questions like this that really inspire people to live in accordance with their desired outcome.

092	Liz	Oh, my face would be more relaxed. I'd be smiling.
093	Elliott	You'd be smiling. Your face would be more relaxed. And how would he know you were . . . you felt good about

this? Like, he would recognize it as different because he hadn't seen it before, I imagine. How would he know you felt good about this difference?

This is powerful. Elliott just changed the question from one of noticing differences to one that helps Liz acknowledge that this change is a good change, a change she is happy with. You can see how Elliott is contributing to the co-construction of this conversation. He inserted the language, through a pre-supposition, that this change was one she felt good about. We have a role to play within these conversations.

094	Liz	Ah, how would he know? You've got me.
095	Elliott	What do you think?

This question is stated so matter-of-factly that there is no way Liz can't continue to think about the answer. Often when meaning is being attributed to details, clients can struggle to articulate something they haven't thought about before. It is our job as SFBT therapists to ask questions that create change. This means that we might have to wait for the change in thought, the change in language, to formulate.

096	Liz	What do I think? How would he know? [*Long pause.*] Probably use his intuition.
097	Elliott	What do you think? He knows you really well. He's watching you and he sees these differences, how would he know, "I've never seen that version of her before, but she seems pleased about it?"

One of the things that Elliott does really well when clients are struggling to come up with a response is to restate the question with more detail. You can see him do that here. He reminds Liz that Bill knows her really well and that he would notice something. When clients "don't know" the answers to the question, you need to restate the question to make it more answerable.

098	Liz	Oh, well again, we'd just go back to my whole body language, facial expression, everything. Yeah.
099	Elliott	Yeah, like the smiling and the relaxing, you said?

Notice that Elliott doesn't try to make this bigger. Elliott is really good at letting the articulated details be good enough. There is a lot of trust in clients when you do this.

100	Liz	Yes. Yes.
101	Elliott	And when you got to the kitchen, where do you find your coffee stuff?

He puts her back into the ongoing desired-outcome description.

102	Liz	On the counter.
103	Elliott	Okay. And what's different about the way you approach the counter when you're this floaty, this pleased, with yourself?

This is a really good example of a question that helps the client articulate difference in the mundane. You notice this conversation hasn't been about anything magical or extraordinary. Liz is simply getting up, dancing a little bit, and now getting coffee. SFBT questions, like this one, should help clients articulate what would be different when the desired outcome intersects with their everyday, mundane life. Again, difference in the mundane is the most likely place change will occur. We should get our clients to tell us about it.

104	Liz	Lack of determination.
105	Elliott	Oh, wow. What would you have instead of determination?

This is an incredible question! When you hear words like determination, *words with positive connotations, we have a tendency to insert our own meaning for these words. Elliott did not get sucked into this potential trap. He took Liz at her word that determination was not useful for her in this minute, something that can be really hard to do! I personally am very impressed by this one!*

Also, Elliott used one of the most important words in SFBT— instead! *Often when you ask clients questions, they will tell you what would be absent in the situation or what wouldn't happen. SFBT is an approach about the presence of the desired outcome. Therefore, you need to know what details would be present. Asking what would be there instead is the very easiest way to find out about the presence of the details. This is a really small detail but a very important one!*

106	Liz	Just . . . just sort of open.
107	Elliott	Just open.
108	Liz	Open, where did that come from? [*She was asking herself that question.*] But anyway, that's what I said.

109   Elliott   How would you know that you had openness instead of determination? Like what would you sense within yourself?

Another good "instead" question.

110   Liz   Lack of tension.

111   Elliott   Oh, wow. Lack of tension. And, and what, what sign would your body give you that the tension was gone and there was openness there in its place?

This is an unusual question for Elliott. He doesn't often ask questions about the person's body. However, this was the question that came to him in the moment. Despite this being an unusual question for him, it gets Liz to start noticing signs that are consistent with the desired outcome—the whole point of this part of the SFBT session. Elliott is still doing his job, even if it's in an unusual way for him.

112   Liz   Relaxation. The feeling of ease.

113   Elliott   Okay. But how would you be aware that the ease was a part of you? You know what I mean? Like what would you be sensing about yourself to tell you the ease was there? Like with tension we get knots in our shoulders. How would you know that the ease was there?

Some might critique Elliott and mention that he introduced problem talk into the session. We are not problem phobic. Often one of the best ways to highlight difference is to mention the problem language that the client used previously—in this case, tension—and then ask about what would be different when the desired outcome was present. Highlighting the contrast is a powerful way to help clients develop the language needed.

114   Liz   [*Long pause.*] I keep thinking of it in terms of lack of, lack of tension, lack of . . .

115   Elliott   Yeah, yeah. And tension gives us clues, doesn't it? Tension lets us know it's there. So what does the ease do to give you a clue that it was there? What do you imagine the ease would do to let you know it's present with you on this day?

You can't tell that Liz has picked up that Elliott keeps asking her the "instead" question. She comments that she keeps thinking about it in the "lack of" perspective. Elliott is so good to acknowledge that this is okay. He says, "Yeah, yeah" with enthusiasm. However, that doesn't dissuade him from his job. He just rephrases his question and asks again. This can be really difficult, especially when Liz is saying she can't answer his question in a different way. He takes that seriously and changes the way he asked his question that will perhaps make it more answerable.

116   Liz   [*Long pause.*] Could you repeat that, please?

117   Elliott   Yeah, yeah. What would the ease do to let you know it was with you at this particular moment?

118   Liz   [*Long pause.*] It would just be a feeling of . . . I want to say contentment.

119   Elliott   Okay. Feeling of contentment. Would you enjoy that?

Elliott's signature checking-in to make sure they are building in the right direction.

120   Liz   Yes.

121   Elliott   Yes. And with this contentment, how would you go about making your coffee then?

Elliott is so skilled at jumping out of the description to get clarification and then jumping right back into the description. He keeps picking up more and more words. Think about all the words he has already learned that are consistent with Liz's desired outcome: free (utterance 4), power (10), centered (16), happy (18), light (40), ecstatic (44), perfect peace (50), not caring what others think (54), floating (72), relaxed (92), lack of determination (104), open (106), and contentment (118). Think about the power that comes when you have this kind of conversation!

122   Liz   Much more easily than when I do it with "get it done."

123   Elliott   Right. And what would be a clue to someone like your husband, who's watched you make coffee ten gazillion times, as he's watching you make this coffee, how would he know you were doing it easily?

This is another difference-in-the-mundane question. Elliott has such a way with these questions.

124   Liz   Probably 'cause I'm not banging cups on the counter.

125   Elliott   Right. Right. So what would you be doing instead then?

Notice the "instead" again!

| 126 | Liz | Everything would be much more gentle. |
| 127 | Elliott | Oh, wow. Okay. So you'd be gentle? |

Simple confirmation question. This serves a great grounding function in conversations.

128	Liz	Yes.
129	Elliott	And how do you take your coffee?
130	Liz	Black.
131	Elliott	Oh, no way?

If you know Elliott at all, you know this just came bursting out of his mouth before he could even think about it. You just have to be yourself!

132	Liz	Yeah! [*Both laugh.*]
133	Elliott	Okay. All right. So you would gently and easily make a cup of black coffee?
134	Liz	Mm-hmm.
135	Elliott	Okay. How long does it take? Are you making an instant coffee? Are you—?
136	Liz	Uck, no!
137	Elliott	No! How do you make it then?
138	Liz	Drip coffee.
139	Elliott	I'm not much of a coffee drinker. How long does that take?

This whole sequence is Elliott allowing Liz to teach him about her world. This helps him know how to ask her questions. These questions also have a secondary benefit of helping the client to feel heard and cared about. Although this isn't the primary function of this conversation, it is a worthwhile side effect!

| 140 | Liz | I'm going to guess about three minutes. |
| 141 | Elliott | So during that three minutes while you're waiting for your black cup of coffee, what would you notice about yourself that would let you know that this ease is still with you as you wait for the three minutes for your drip coffee to be prepared? |

Elliott has done it once again. He took a little detour to learn about the coffee so that he could infuse those details into this question. Notice the blackness of the coffee is present, the three minutes is present, and the drip preparation is present. He is picking up all those details so that he can ask this question. The details make the question richer.

Also, he went back several utterances (into the 120s) and picked up the word ease *again. You have to be this good at remembering the details in order for the session to look and sound like this.*

142	Liz	That's too funny. What just came to me is that I would be ignoring the coffee pot. Normally I'm going, "Dammit, get done!" [*Both laugh.*]
143	Elliott	Really?
144	Liz	Yeah.
145	Elliott	So as you ignore the coffee pot, what do you imagine you would be thinking about instead?

Do you see how every answer Liz provides, Elliott accepts wholeheartedly?

One of the other really profound things he keeps doing is changing the medium of his questions. He has asked about feelings, he has asked about doing (or actions), and now he is asking about thoughts. This is a really comprehensive consideration of all the various aspects of Liz. Each of these components would be affected by the presence of the desired outcome.

146	Liz	[*Very long pause.*] Gratitude.
147	Elliott	And what do you imagine is the first thing you'd be grateful about?

Here Elliott inserts the word first *again.*

148	Liz	The coffee making itself.
149	Elliott	Okay. Then what?

This is the classic "What else?" question without using those exact words.

150	Liz	More gratitude?
151	Elliott	What else would you be grateful about? Three minutes is a big while.

Again, when clients are taken off guard or don't understand the question, providing more detail (e.g., "Three minutes is a big while") helps to jog their memory about where we are in the description.

152	Liz	Oh, okay. I'm drawing an absolute blank on that one.
153	Elliott	What do you think? What other things might give you some feelings of gratitude?

Elliott doesn't do anything except ask the question again. He doesn't bail Liz out when she says she is drawing a blank, and he doesn't try to offer suggestions about what she could be grateful for. He trusts completely that she can answer these questions. After all, someone with power, centeredness, and contentment doesn't need a clinician to provide them with answers!

154	Liz	Well, gratitude popped into mind, cause I'm doing a thirty-day gratitude exercise right now.
155	Elliott	Yeah, yeah.
156	Liz	So that's at the front of my mind.
157	Elliott	Those types of challenge are pretty cool, huh?
158	Liz	Well, are they ever! What else would I be?
159	Elliott	Yeah, what else would you have gratitude about?

You can see that Elliott just keeps asking the same question until he gets an answer.

160	Liz	Oh, the gratitude. I'm finding that there's so much to be grateful for. I'm almost at the end of the time. And the longer it goes on, the more I realize how much we have to be grateful for. Things like just having the air in here, the heat on, a rug on the floor, a couch to sit on, a roof over my head, food whenever I want it.
161	Elliott	Yeah. So how different would it be for during that three minutes, while the coffee was making itself, for you to be thinking about the air and the couch and the home and "I have all of the things to be grateful for," versus saying, "Dammit, hurry up, coffee." How different would that be?

Elliott did his job really nicely here. Even though Liz was talking about the current gratitude exercise she is working on, Elliott brought out those things that she is grateful for and the thoughts of gratitude into the description of the desired outcome. This is a really clear example of not getting by on good things at the expense of paying attention to the best thing! Your job is a desired-outcome description, and you might have to work to piece the puzzle together in order to do your job.

162 Liz A hundred percent.

163 Elliott A hundred percent. And would you be pleased to be spending that three minutes with a sense of gratitude?

You can see that there is a pattern that is being created. New details are provided, Elliott asks about the level of difference, then checks in to see if Liz is pleased with the difference. This pattern is setting up a reality that Liz has created with language that is completely different from her previous reality.

164 Liz Totally.

165 Elliott Totally. Okay. And after the three minutes was done, what would you do next? Where do you go to enjoy your coffee?

166 Liz Right now, I sit outside and smoke.

167 Elliott You sit outside. So where would you go enjoy this coffee on this day, when you're at your absolute best with all this control that the five- and six-year-old version of you absolutely had?

This is a powerful example of the use of language. Do you see how Elliott preserved the "sitting outside," while dropping the "smoking"? When clients give you a choice about what to pick up and what to leave behind, you should choose to leave behind the details that are inconsistent with the desired outcome.

Liz is free to say anything she wants (every answer is the correct answer). Elliott has the responsibility to make this answer constructive within the conversation. In this case, you can see that Elliott just reminds Liz that they are talking about a different kind of day, but he doesn't do that in a condescending way or in a way that he argues with Liz about not smoking. This is a straightforward but powerful question that is constructed very carefully!

| 168 | Liz | Oh, okay. Well, I didn't really drink coffee at five or six. I would be sitting in comfort inside and enjoying my coffee. |

| 169 | Elliott | Okay. So where inside, on this morning with that inner person taking control, where would you enjoy your coffee? |

Elliott is so good at continually infusing Liz's previous desired-outcome language into each question. Here he mentions control *again. Do you see that the mundane coffee drinking becomes something very different when someone who is taking control does it?*

| 170 | Liz | On the couch, in front of the fireplace. |

| 171 | Elliott | In front of the fireplace. On the couch. Okay. And as you were walking over to the couch in front of the fireplace, what would you notice about the way you were heading over there that would let you know, *This is me at my absolute best, at my most controlled*? |

There is another presupposition built into this question. "What would you notice about the way you were heading over there . . . ." assumes that Liz would notice something. However, Elliott then adds the desired-outcome words such as "absolute best" and "most controlled" that qualify the answer that Liz can give. This is a prime example of co-constructing a description that is consistent with the desired outcome.

| 172 | Liz | My footsteps would be softer. I wouldn't be, sort of, marching, which I have been known to do. So my footsteps would be softer, and I would just be feeling much more at ease. |

| 173 | Elliott | Would you really? Okay. And how would you pick the place on the couch? How would you go about selecting where to sit? |

This shows the level of difference you are looking for in a solution focused session. In SFBT, we believe that the desired outcome being present would positively impact everything—in this case, from the way Liz walks to the way she makes silly decisions about where to sit on the couch. Because the desired outcome completely changes Liz, it completely impacts everything she does. Because she is different, everything she does is different!

174	Liz	I just sit.
175	Elliott	How many options do you have?
176	Liz	On the couch, I have two.
177	Elliott	Ah, so you just pick one half, and as you're sitting there enjoying your coffee, what's the very first thing you might notice?

To be honest, I'm a little surprised that Elliott let her off the hook. He simply took that she would choose a seat. Typically he would wait for her to articulate which seat she chose. However, I imagine that she won't be able to look at the couch next time without thinking about the decision she needs to make.

178	Liz	How good the coffee is.
179	Elliott	Do you enjoy this coffee?
180	Liz	I do.
181	Elliott	What brand is it?
182	Liz	It's the dark French roast.
183	Elliott	And it's just black. You haven't put anything in it?
184	Liz	No. Nope, I'm sorry. I lied. I put cardamom in it.
185	Elliott	Cardamom. I don't even know what that is.
186	Liz	Oh, it neutralizes the acidity of coffee.
187	Elliott	Gotcha. Well maybe I should do that. I don't like coffee because there's too much acid.

This whole sequence really highlights that Elliott doesn't try to be a therapist. He really just tries to be himself, and therapy gets done. I heard a great quote from Eve Lipchik that seems to apply really nicely here: "Remember you are a human first, a therapist second, and a solution focused therapist third." Elliott really lives in that human space.

188	Liz	Ah, try it with cardamom. It's great!
189	Elliott	So as you're sitting there enjoying your cardamom coffee and you're just noticing how good it is, what else might you notice?

And then he gets right back to the task at hand. The description continues.

190	Liz	How fortunate I am to be able to do that.

| 191 | Elliott | Oh. How different would that be for you to have that thought that *I'm so fortunate to be able to do this*? |

This is another unique way that Elliott seems to use the concept of difference. In this question, he is asking Liz to comment on the level of difference that she would be experiencing. I don't know another therapist who asks this kind of question. However, since this is a difference-oriented approach, this kind of question really serves to highlight that difference is really in the focal point of the conversation.

192	Liz	How different is that?
193	Elliott	Yes, ma'am.
194	Liz	I don't know. I've been thinking a lot lately.
195	Elliott	How much like a five- or six-year-old, who didn't care that much, would that feel like? If this version of you was sitting there, how much would that feel congruent to that person?

This is a beautiful question that alters the previous question, based on the feedback from Liz in utterance 194. Elliott moves from asking about how different that would be to how congruent it would be to Liz's five- or six-year-old confident self. This highlights that he was trying to make a connection back to the desired outcome in the previous question, but it fell flat. This is a much clearer, precise question that links the conversation back to the desired outcome. Elliott is so good at listening to Liz and accommodating his questions to match her needs.

| 196 | Liz | [*Long pause.*] I'm not getting anything. |
| 197 | Elliott | Then what's the next clue you would notice that would remind you that you're still that person? |

Again, Elliott is willing to change his question to make it more applicable/answerable for Liz. However, you can see that even in changing the question, he is still keeping the new question consistent with the desired outcome. His role in the conversation didn't change, even though he is responding to the needs of the client.

198	Liz	The ease and comfort I'd be feeling.
199	Elliott	That seems to be . . . You use that several times, like this ease and comfort.
200	Liz	Really?

201   Elliott   Yeah. The ease and comfort would be important to you, it seems like.

202   Liz   Yes.

203   Elliott   And different perhaps, it feels like.

This interchange is really interesting. Liz seemed really surprised to hear that she had mentioned ease and comfort several times. It is obvious to us as we read this transcript that "ease" especially is there over and over. This highlights that clients may not consciously be aware of the changes they are making, especially at the language level. However, it is clear to see that Liz does acknowledge that this is important to her and that it is different from what she was experiencing before coming to the session.

204   Liz   Yes.

205   Elliott   And so what would be the next way you might notice this ease and comfort were a part of you as you were sitting on the couch, enjoying your cardamom coffee?

206   Liz   I would be able to fully accept it.

207   Elliott   And how would you know you accepted it? That's an interesting thing.

This last phrase, "That's an interesting thing," is another unusual comment from Elliott. You can see that he rarely inserts his own thoughts in a session. This is one of the few times.

208   Liz   How would I know it? When I didn't think, *Oh my God, what's happened?*

209   Elliott   Right.

210   Liz   Without thinking, *Is it going to go away?*

211   Elliott   Right. So what might you be thinking instead that would feel like, *I'm accepting it?*

This is another great example of the "instead" question. It hardly seems like Elliott is asking the same question he asked before. Because we are at a different part of the session, and because the language used at this point in the session is different, this question really feels like a different question.

212   Liz   [*Long pause.*] I would be thinking of other things. I wouldn't even be considering it.

213   Elliott   Right.

214   Liz   Yeah.

215   Elliott   And what's the type of stuff, Liz, that you might think about?

This question just seems so logical and simple. However, think about what he is really asking: "When you are different, when you are in control, when you have ease, when you have comfort, what kinds of things would you be thinking about?" This is a really powerful question.

216   Liz   God, horses, cats, birds, being in the forest, being at the ocean, kayaking.

217   Elliott   Are those all things you enjoy?

Just another check-in here. Liz has just taught Elliott new language.

218   Liz   Yes.

219   Elliott   Okay. Do you own cats, horses, and . . . ?

220   Liz   Not now. I'm animal-less.

221   Elliott   Animal-less. Okay. So how different would it be for you to be sitting there thinking about all these things that you would enjoy? Cats, horses, animals, birds, kayaking?

Elliott asks another "how different" question. Again, this kind of question helps him know how much attention to spend on these things.

222   Liz   Ah, great! How different?

223   Elliott   Yes, ma'am, how different?

224   Liz   Yes, because I don't think of it much anymore, because I don't want to be missing what I don't have.

225   Elliott   So as you thought about it on this day, instead of missing it, how would you describe that feeling?

This "instead" question serves another really important function. Elliott picked up on the fact that when Liz thought about these things during a time when she was relaxed, in control, and at ease, that these thoughts would be different. Even though the thoughts are about the same things (horses, animals, kayaking, etc.) that might have made her miss them before, when she thinks about them in this state she would have a different experience. Highlighting this difference creates a very powerful shift in the meaning of these thoughts. This is the difference in the mundane again.

| 226 | Liz | Instead of missing it? |

227 Elliott Yes, ma'am.

228 Liz How would I describe the feeling? Emptiness.

229 Elliott Emptiness. And would this be like a good emptiness because there's no missing it, or a bad emptiness?

This clarifying question is important because Elliott can't attribute meaning to the answer without the help of Liz.

230 Liz It would be a bad emptiness, because I would be missing it.

231 Elliott You would be missing it. Okay. But if you weren't missing it [*Liz: Yep*], because you were at your very best and you were thinking about these things you enjoy, what would you be doing instead, as you thought about these things?

This is a really hard question to ask! Some people might say that Elliott just changed the meaning of what Liz said. She said she would be missing these things, and Elliott just said she wouldn't be. To understand this, you have to go all the way back to utterance 215. Liz mentioned that she would be thinking about these things when she was accepting the ease that she was feeling. She had a moment of realization, but then the conversation turned a bit.

I would argue that because Elliott has been talking about the desired outcome the entire session, he knows that Liz linked these things and thoughts to the desired outcome. Therefore, even though she is now saying that she would be missing these things, Elliott can know that he can turn that around because she acknowledged previously that this was part of the experience of ease.

When you track the language really carefully, you can see that Elliott is going back to the first way Liz mentioned these thoughts, rather than focusing on the way she is describing them now. This is very tricky! However, if you know you have stayed really close to the desired outcome, you can do things like ask this question.

232 Liz I'm not missing them.

233   Elliott   Yeah. You're still thinking about them . . .

234   Liz   Yeah. I'd be remembering all the wonderful times we had and all the things we did.

235   Elliott   Okay. And instead of missing it, what do you call that?

This is a really Elliott question. Identifying things by name makes them easier to refer to later on in the conversation. This naming isn't for narrative-therapy purposes. Instead, it is about having usable language to work with in the ongoing co-construction.

236   Liz   Fond memories.

237   Elliott   Fond memories. And how different would it be for you to be thinking about these wonderful things with fondness instead of emptiness or missing them?

Here is another difference question. The conversation has gotten to a place where they are on the same page again. They are back to talking about life in the presence of the desired outcome, where the same everyday experience would mean something very different. This is how change happens through language.

238   Liz   Wow! That would be a big shift, actually. Yeah. Very different.

239   Elliott   Would you enjoy that?

240   Liz   Yes.

241   Elliott   Would you be pleased about thinking about these things with fondness?

Another grounding sequence that is based on satisfaction with where the conversation has gone.

242   Liz   Instead of missing them? Yes.

243   Elliott   Yes, ma'am. Okay. And how long do you think you would sit on the couch by the fireplace and enjoy these memories?

Again, you can notice a pattern of Elliott asking for confirmation that he is following and understanding—he is grounding correctly. Then he asks a question that uses the details of the future-of-the-outcome conversation to reorient Liz back into the account of what would be happening.

| 244 | Liz | I'm going to say a maximum of ten minutes 'cause that's how long it takes for me to drink a coffee. |
| 245 | Elliott | Fast coffee drinker. It takes me forty-seven hours. [*Both laugh.*] After the ten minutes, what would you do next? |

Again, you can see Elliott's humor here. That humor doesn't get in the way of the ongoing description, however.

| 246 | Liz | And then I'm assuming this is literal, so I would go and rinse out my coffee cup. |
| 247 | Elliott | It is literal, yes. And what's different about the way you are heading over to rinse out the coffee cup? |

I'm sure you know by now, but this is a continuation of inquiring about difference, because everything is different about the way Liz does everything.

| 248 | Liz | I'm still just perfectly comfortable and not worried about other things. |
| 249 | Elliott | Right. So what would you be thinking about then? Instead of worrying, what might you be doing? |

It is interesting to see how many times Elliott asks Liz what she would be doing "instead." She never seems annoyed nor does she insinuate that she feels that this question is redundant. Knowing about difference is clearly the focus of this session.

250	Liz	I don't know. It's not very far. Not really time to think.
251	Elliott	Oh, you think [*snaps his finger three times*] that fast?
252	Liz	I know. Just trying to divert you here. [*Both laugh.*]
253	Elliott	Not easy to do.
254	Liz	Yeah. [*Both laugh.*] What would I be thinking? Oh, yes. What I had to do after that.
255	Elliott	Right. And what's the typical thing you might have to do, Liz?

I really like the inclusion of the word typical *here. This miracle day doesn't change anything about the day; it only changes Liz and how she interacts with the day.*

| 256 | Liz | Put on my shoes and go out for a walk. |

257   Elliott   Really? And what's different about the way you take your walk when you're free and in control and in power? What's different about the way you take your walk?

It probably doesn't surprise you to see this question at this point in the session. The desired-outcome language is there, the emphasis on difference is there, and the current language being used by Liz is there. All the elements of a good SFBT question are present.

258   Liz   Well, actually, we had a glimpse of that, so I can actually use it. I go with some neighborhood people and their dogs, and it's quite an interesting group. At my best, I'm able to walk and just be totally aware of their energies but not accepting any of the toxicity.

It is interesting to note that Liz is now identifying the differences she has been talking about, but now it is consistent with things that have already happened. It is often the case that, as people describe their desired outcome, they realize that at least some pieces or signs of the description have already happened before. Liz is highlighting one of these "instances" of success that has already happened.

It is also interesting to note that Liz used the phrase "at my best." This is the first time she has used this phrase. Elliott was actually the one who introduced this into the conversation (see utterances 85, 91, and others), and he has used it several times, but now Liz is also using it. This is evidence that language is being co-constructed.

259   Elliott   Really?

260   Liz   Yes.

261   Elliott   So you'd be aware of the energy but not accepting their toxicity?

Another grounding question that confirms he heard and understood correctly.

262   Liz   Yes. There's one that's quite toxic.

263   Elliott   Okay. And what would you do instead of accepting the toxicity? What would you be doing?

Some might be alarmed that Elliott asked a question that led to "problem talk." However, it is vital to help our clients to feel heard and understood. If we ignore statements that include problems, our clients will feel invalidated. Elliott is

> *a master of acknowledging facts like this but then switching it back to the desired-outcome description with an "instead" question. Can you see why "instead" is one of the most important words in SFBT?*

264	Liz	I actually usually start with one of the other people in a lighthearted bantering manner, and it spreads to the group.

265	Elliott	And so somehow you spread lightheartedness and this bantering as opposed to the other person spreading toxicity?

> *Notice that because they are now talking about something that has happened previously, rather than a hypothetical situation in the future, the tense of the language has shifted to the present tense. They are now talking about changes/situations that are consistent with the desired outcome that has and is currently happening. Change is happening in this session through the language!*

266	Liz	Yes.

267	Elliott	Okay. And how would they know that you were somehow the most controlled, most free, most powerful version of yourself that they had yet seen?

> *Elliott is so quick with these presuppositions. He assumes that the neighbors will notice the pieces or characteristics of the desired outcome. There is confidence in this question.*

268	Liz	I don't think they're aware of it at all.

269	Elliott	But they still might pick something up, wouldn't they?

> *There is persistence in this question—the underlying belief that, when Liz is different, others will notice, and is ever-present in the work Elliott does.*

270	Liz	All they know is that the energy has changed.

271	Elliott	How would they know?

> *Elliott's previous persistence paid off. Liz was able to come up with an answer (without much difficulty, actually). This question from Elliott allows Liz to take credit for the change. Liz attributed the change to a change in the energy. However, Elliott can ask questions that help highlight that Liz has something to do with this change.*

272	Liz	Because they're laughing and talking and being insane, instead of . . .
273	Elliott	Okay. And would you be pleased that they were picking up this energy from you and that there was more laughing and talking and those types of things?

There is a very subtle shift in Elliott's language here. Do you see that he gave all the credit for the change in energy to Liz? He added, "this energy from you." Liz does not disagree with him about this addition, because she previously mentioned that she deliberately tried to change the mood to lighthearted banter. It is hard to disagree when you supplied the previous details! Liz not only doesn't disagree; she also agrees whole-heartedly—see below.

274	Liz	Totally. Yes.
275	Elliott	You would. How would they know they were walking with a woman who was pleased about the impact she was having on others?

Notice how Elliott is giving Liz the credit more and more, and Liz is receiving it more and more. This is a masterful use of language by Elliott.

276	Liz	Ah, just keep up the lightheartedness.
277	Elliott	Yeah. But, you know, what would they see? What would be there, as they looked at you? How would they know they were looking at someone who was pleased with the way she was doing things on this day?

It is common for people to try to attribute difference to whim, circumstances, luck, or just chance. Elliott is co-constructing a reality where Liz can take credit for the difference.

278	Liz	Yeah. You know, it's a hard one. I really don't believe they are aware of that.
279	Elliott	Aware of which part?
280	Liz	Anybody. How anybody's energy has changed and is affecting others.
281	Elliott	So you're not sure they would catch it.

This sequence is really interesting because Liz seems sure that her neighbors wouldn't catch the difference. One of the things I wonder, as an outside observer, is if there is a bit of confusion happening between Elliott and Liz. Liz seems to be talking about a situation that has already happened (since she mentioned this happened previously). Elliott seems to be talking about an event in the future where this similar situation might happen again. Liz seems to be answering that her neighbors wouldn't notice, because she doesn't think they did notice anything different. However, if Elliott could take a second and say, "If this similar interaction were to happen again, what do you think they would notice?" it might make this question a little easier to answer.

Please know that I'm not criticizing Elliott at all. This is a very subtle nuance and would be very difficult to catch when a conversation is happening in real time. As therapists, we all have these kinds of things happen in our sessions, but we aren't all willing to put our work out there for the whole world to see. This sequence shows that sometimes we have difficulty grounding with our clients about certain details. When this happens, it might be worth stopping for a second to think about what might be happening at the language level.

282	Liz	I am sure they don't.
283	Elliott	Okay. If they did, what might they catch?

There it is! Elliott completely bought that "they DON'T notice" from Liz. However, he just corrected the miscommunication by asking about if they DID notice. That's all it takes. One small adjustment and the conversation is back on track.

284	Liz	Oh my gosh. If they did. Okay. Let's strip away their personalities. [*Both laugh.*]
285	Elliott	If they did, what might they touch upon?
286	Liz	They would see the . . . They would just see the . . . the tempered and ease and feel of it.
287	Elliott	Hmm, okay. Right, right. And how long is your walk? Where do you go?

Elliott got the answer, so that part of the conversation has been completed. (They arrived back at the best hopes.) He can now move the conversation on to the next moment of the description.

288	Liz	Oh, it's usually about half an hour. And we just take a short path through the woods.

289   Elliott   Oh, through the woods. What would you notice as you walked through the woods that would fit with someone who is at ease?

290   Liz   Oh, the beauty. There's a mountain just shortly in the distance. In the winter, the sun just glistens off the snow. This time of year, the colors, the fir trees. Oh, yeah.

291   Elliott   Really? And would you be enjoying this beauty? Would you be taking this beauty in?

Here's that pattern again. He asks about a detail and checks to see if Liz is pleased by it.

292   Liz   Absolutely.

293   Elliott   Okay. And what would you notice about yourself, though, that would let you know that you were out here with freedom and control and really taking in the beauty?

This is another really important question. Elliott can't let the description just be about noticing details in the surroundings; the miracle doesn't change those things. Instead, Elliott has to make sure that he connects the changes back to the desired outcome. What does Liz notice about herself as she is taking in this beauty? This can be such an easy thing to forget in the moment, especially when the details provided are this magnificent. However, your job is to not get distracted by the details but home in on the details that are consistent with the best hopes. Elliott is so good at remembering this from the beginning of the session right to the very end.

294   Liz   I have to go back to the sense of ease again.

295   Elliott   Yeah, that seems to be a very common thing when you have this control and power that you are talking about. This ease.

296   Liz   Ah, okay.

Again, Liz seems a little surprised by this observation by Elliott.

297   Elliott   Excellent. Well, Liz, I think we're running out of time. I want to invite you to do two things, if you don't mind.

298   Liz   Yes.

299   Elliott   I'm so fascinated by the word *ease*. You used it a lot.

300	Liz	I'm going to have to spend some time on that.
301	Elliott	I would. I want you to just notice how often the ease shows up in your life. Maybe it will be a moment standing by the coffee pot, as the coffee gets prepared and you're having a moment of gratitude, who knows? But I want you to kind of be an "ease detective" for a bit, if you don't mind.
302	Liz	Interesting. I will do that.
303	Elliott	And then the second thing: I'd love to hear how things are going. Would you mind sending me an e-mail?
304	Liz	Absolutely. Yes.
305	Elliott	Yeah. Cool.

It is a little uncommon for Elliott to give a homework assignment. However, when he does, it looks similar to this. He will ask people to notice the details that are consistent with what they mentioned during the session. Anything beyond that would violate the client's autonomy and agency.

The end of the session is often brief and succinct like this. An SFBT therapist tries very hard to not undo any of the work that has been done during the session.

Appendix C

Glossary

Closing: How an SFBT session is wrapped up. Typically the focus of this part of the conversation is to ensure that the description from earlier in the conversation is not undone. Most commonly a closing includes thanking the client for contributing to the conversation and letting them know they are welcome to return for another session if they feel that doing so would be beneficial. All other conversation is kept to a minimum. Clinicians avoid giving a summary of the conversation, making suggestions for future steps, and/or providing compliments to the client, even if the compliments are accurate.

Co-construction: The maximum collaboration of the client's agency, which is expressed through the client's language, with the expertise of the clinician to structure a therapy session around the client's desired outcome.

Description: The detailed explanation of the transformation/desired outcome being present in the client's life.

Desired outcome (best hopes): The transformation the client is pursuing in therapy. The best hopes is one question that can be used to begin the conversation with clients about said transformation.

The diamond: An SFBT framework that details how to conceptualize the SFBT approach, its principles, theoretical orientation, strategies, and techniques clinicians use to help clients co-construct their desired outcome and related details.

History of the outcome: A conversation, which is a description pathway, that includes details related to the transformation/desired outcome that is focused on sometime in the past, most commonly when the desired outcome was most significantly present.

Preferred future: A conversation, which is a description pathway, that includes details related to the transformation/desired outcome that is focused on sometime in the future, most commonly the day after the current conversation.

Presupposition: A linguistic tool that makes an assumption that is related to the conversation in which the truth of the assumption is taken for granted by the speaker.

Resource talk: A conversation, which is a description pathway, that includes strengths, qualities, characteristics, and skills that a person possesses to achieve a transformation/desired outcome.

Scaling: A conversation that includes numeric representations from 0 to 10, in which 10 represents the complete presence of the transformation/desired outcome, and 0 represents the complete absence of the transformation/desired outcome.

Solution focused brief therapy: A therapeutic approach developed by Steve de Shazer, Insoo Kim Berg, and colleagues. SFBT is based on a co-constructed conversation between a client (or clients) and a clinician that is focused on identifying a desired outcome of the client and developing a description of the changes or differences that would be present when the desired outcome is present in the client's life.

SFBT Resources

Websites

- The Solution Focused Universe page: thesfu.com
- Elliott's page: elliottconnie.com
- A research page in development: solutionfocusedbrieftherapy.com

App

- SFBT Electronic Health Record: app.solutionfocusednotes.com

Social Media Handles

Facebook

- Elliott Connie
- Adam Froerer
- Solution Focused Universe

Instagram

- @elliottspeaks
- @adam.froerer
- @thesolutionfocuseduniverse
- @solutionfocusednotes

Twitter

- @ElliottSpeaks
- @AFroerer
- @thesfu_

LinkedIn

- Elliott Connie
- Adam Froerer

YouTube

- Elliott Connie

Books

- *Solution-Focused Brief Therapy with Clients Managing Trauma*, by Adam Froerer, Jacqui von Cziffra-Bergs, Johnny Kim, and Elliott Connie
- *The Art of Solution Focused Therapy*, by Elliott Connie and Linda Metcalf
- *Solution Building in Couples Therapy*, by Elliott Connie
- *The Solution Focused Marriage: 5 Simple Habits That Will Bring Out the Best in Your Relationship*, by Elliott Connie

Reference List

American Psychiatric Association. (2013). *Diagnostic and statistical manual of mental disorders* (5th ed.). https://doi.org/10.1176/appi. books.9780890425596

American Psychological Association. (2012). *Research shows psychotherapy is effective but underutilized* [Press release]. https://www.apa.org/news /press/releases/2012/08/psychotherapy-effective#

Dryden, W. (2018). The modal number of therapy sessions internationally is 'one', and the majority of people who attend for one session are satisfied. In W. Dryden (Ed.), *Single-session therapy*. Routledge, London.

Froerer, A. S., Walker, C. R., & Lange, P. Solution focused brief therapy presuppositions: A comparison of 1.0 and 2.0 SFBT approaches. [Manuscript submitted for publication].

Madan, C. R., Scott, S. M. E., & Kensinger, E. A. (2019). Positive emotion enhances association-memory. *Emotion, 19*(4). https://doi.org/10.1037 /emo0000465.

McKergow, M. (2016). SFBT 2.0: The next generation of solution-focused brief therapy has already arrived. *Journal of Solution Focused Practices, 2*(2).

Index

Acknowledgments

This book could never have happened without the help and support of many people. First, we would like to thank Reid Tracy for believing in this book and taking a risk on us. Without your vision about what is possible for changing the way we approach mental health, this book would have been a nonstarter. Thank you for seeing the vision and trusting us with creating this project.

Next we would like to thank Jeff Walker. Thank you for seeing something in me (Elliott) that I didn't even see in myself at the time. Thank you for helping me push beyond what I thought was possible and for sharing your wisdom and insight with me.

We would like to send a special thank you to Melody Guy, our editor at Hay House, for maintaining an integrity for this process. Thank you for listening to our vision and for making it happen. You gave us invaluable feedback and immeasurable freedom to do what we thought was important. Thank you for walking the line between expert and guide. Your help, support, and encouragement made this journey pleasant and meaningful.

A special thank you must be given to Kathryn Purdie for being absolutely amazing! Thank you for dedicating your time and talents to help make this project what it is today. Quite literally this project would never have seen the light of day without your help and support! It was a pleasure to work with you on this project from day one. We consider it divine intervention that you came into our lives at the perfect moment. Beyond the contribution of your unique skills to this project, we are so grateful just to call you a friend. Thank you!

We obviously need to thank Steve de Shazer, Insoo Kim Berg, Yvonne Dolan, Eve Lipchik, and the other founding members of this approach. Without their courage and pioneering efforts, this approach would not have been a part of our lives. We also want to thank Chris Iveson, Evan George, and Harvey Ratner for teaching us that we could do SFBT in our own way. Thank you for guiding and mentoring us along our solution focused journey. We wouldn't be where we are today without you!

It would have been impossible for us to dedicate so much time and energy to completing this project without the help and support of our team at The Solution Focused Universe. Thank you, Anna Francis, for running the company so skillfully. Your leadership and dedication to the community is outstanding. Thank you for compensating for us in many ways, but especially as we worked on this project. Thank you for all the encouragement, support, and motivating energy to complete this project! Thanks for bringing comic relief when we needed it! Thank you to Helen Holman and Taylor Tyler for working tirelessly to make the brand well loved and for growing interest in our message. And thank you to Cecil Walker for engaging in endless conversations about the details of this approach and for stimulating new ideas and understanding. You have each made meaningful contributions to this book and it wouldn't be what it is without your support. Thank you!

Finally, to Carmesia, Madison, and David, and to Becca, Rachel, Toby, and Julia, thank you for loving us and supporting each of our outlandish ideas. Thank you for treating us like we are capable of completing this enormous task, especially on the hard days. Thank you for your unconditional love and acceptance. We love you and hope we make you proud!

About the Authors

Elliott Connie is an accomplished psychotherapist and a leading voice in the field of solution focused brief therapy. He's been credentialed since 2006 and been in private practice since 2008. He has a bachelor's in psychology and a master's of science in professional counselling. He has worked alongside some of the most prominent figures in the SFBT field. Additionally, Elliott has lectured all over the United States as well as internationally, in places such as the United Kingdom, Russia, India and Australia.

Adam Froerer is one of the leading SFBT researchers and trainers. He has a bachelor's degree in psychology, a master's of education in marriage and family therapy, and a doctorate of philosophy also in marriage and family therapy. He worked as a university professor for 11 years, training marriage and family therapists and clinical psychologists. Adam has had the privilege of working with amazing clinicians, trainers, and researchers from around the globe.

Adam and Elliott founded The Solution Focused Universe (SFU), the largest solution focused training institute in the world. Through live and online courses and trainings, they train approximately 15,000 individuals annually. The SFU also houses the largest library of solution focused training material available. Because this work is so important to them, and because they want to make sure this approach gets out to the whole world, they are also behind the training institute that provides the most free content in the world. **www.solutionfocusedbrieftherapy.com**

Hay House Titles of Related Interest

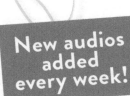